"In the depths of a desperate struggle
with alcoholism, I found a medicine, baclofen, that
both freed me of all craving for alcohol and resolved the
underlying disorder, overwhelming anxiety that made
me vulnerable to addiction. By completely suppressing
my addiction, baclofen saved my life."

— *Olivier Ameisen, MD*, The End of My Addiction

THE END OF ALCOHOL ADDICTION

Baclofen, a New Tool in the Fight Against Alcoholism

Mathis Heydtmann, MD, PhD

Jonathan Chick, MD, MA, MBChB, MPhil, DSc

Renaud de Beaurepaire, MD

Antonio Mirijello, MD

Lorenzo Leggio, MD, PhD, MSc

Giovanni Addolorato, MD

Mehdi Farokhnia, MD

Philippe Jaury, MD

Edited by Mary Van Beusekom, ELS, MWC

SUNRISE
River Press

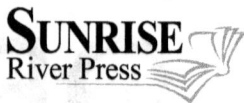

SUNRISE River Press

Sunrise River Press
838 Lake Street South
Forest Lake, MN 55025
Phone: 651-277-1400 or 800-895-4585
Fax: 651-277-1203
www.sunriseriverpress.com

Edit by Mary Van Beusekom

ISBN 978-1-934716-63-2
Item No. SRP663

Library of Congress Cataloging-in-Publication Data

Names: Heydtmann, Mathis, author.
Title: Baclofen : a new tool in the fight against alcoholism / Mathis
  Heydtmann, MD, PhD [and 9 others].
Description: Forest Lake, MN : Sunrise River Press, 2017. | Includes
  bibliographical references and index.
Identifiers: LCCN 2017005682 | ISBN 9781934716632
Subjects: LCSH: Muscle relaxants. | Alcoholism.
Classification: LCC RM312 .H49 2017 | DDC 615.7/73–dc23
LC record available at https://lccn.loc.gov/2017005682

Printed in USA
10 9 8 7 6 5 4 3 2 1

Contents

Introduction

Mathis Heydtmann, MD, PhD, Consultant Hepatologist and
Gastroenterologist, RAH Paisley, Scotland

Scott was 54 years old when he was first admitted to our hospital with severe alcoholic liver disease. He was a hard-working family man and had managed to hold down his job at the airport despite his long-standing problems with alcohol. As a teenager, Scott used to binge on alcohol almost every day with his friends. He described himself at that time as anxious, particularly regarding social situations; thus, when he drank with his friends, it eased his anxiety and it was easier for him to speak within the group. When he started to work, at first as a baggage handler at the airport, he stopped drinking during the week. However, his social life continued to center on drinking with his friends over the weekends, and this did not change even when he married and had 2 children.

After an accident at work when he was in his 40s, he stopped drinking and decided to stay away from alcohol. He managed to do this for about 1 year despite having strong alcohol cravings at first. However, when his mother died 8 years ago, Scott started to drink more and more often, including during the week because it helped him sleep. He tried to stop drinking again 5 years ago when his marriage almost broke up, but quitting did not work because he had severe alcohol cravings. On several occasions, he went into delirium tremens, a set of severe signs and symptoms of alcohol withdrawal, and had to be admitted to the hospital for detox.

A few weeks after he left the hospital, he began drinking again, and his family doctor referred him to his local medical alcohol abuse team. The team gave him prescriptions for the drugs acamprosate and disulfiram, but he continued to drink alcohol.

Over time, Scott had several short hospital admissions for injuries, skin infections, and alcohol withdrawal syndrome. Throughout that time, he wanted badly to stop drinking, but he could not. He said he didn't even like the taste of alcohol, but over the years, he needed increasing amounts of higher-proof (stronger) alcohol to get the same effect and stave off alcohol withdrawal symptoms.

The great burden of alcoholism

Scott is typical of the people with alcohol use disorder whom doctors see in their general practices and in hospitals every day in every specialty, including medical and surgical specialties. The number of patients with alcohol use disorders is particularly high in Scotland, where hospital admissions for alcoholic liver disease are higher than in other parts of Western Europe, including the rest of the United Kingdom. In Scotland, there were nearly 35,000 alcohol-related hospital admissions in 2015, according to National Services Scotland.[1]

The worldwide burden of alcoholism on the individuals, their families, and society is enormous. People with alcohol use disorders tend to see their family doctor often, miss time at work, get into problems with the law, have financial difficulties, alienate their family and friends, and may be admitted to the hospital several times per year. Alcohol contributes to such health problems as heart disease, stroke, liver disease, brain damage, pancreatitis, and cancer, as well as such societal problems as suicide, domestic violence, accidents, and crime.

Although we have some understanding of addictions such as the addiction to alcohol, there is still a significant unmet need to help this patient group recover. Certainly, this patient group is not easy to treat because, as part of the addictive personality, these patients often have chaotic lifestyles and do not prioritize their health as much as they should. This leads them to miss routine doctor appointments such as follow-up and screening visits and to neglect their health in general. In addition, they often have poor nutrition and poor dental care; and these are just a few of the most common problems. When addiction becomes a priority, people tend to do things that they would not normally do, and principles and values that used to be important, including honesty, become not as important as being able to satisfy the addiction.

The other issue is that medical, addiction, and psychiatric services in hospitals as well as in the community are often set up separately in silos, with the specialty in mind rather than the patient at the center of their care, where they need to be. Because people with alcohol addiction usually have needs that are far too complex for any one specialty or person to deal with, they are at risk for "falling between the cracks" and having their needs go unmet. Addiction in general and alcohol addiction in particular is a massive problem worldwide, with 3.3 million deaths every year from the harmful use of alcohol and 5.1% of the global burden of disease and injury attributable to alcohol.[2]

As with other substances with a potential for addiction, alcohol has been consumed by humans for thousands of years. Whereas for many addictive behaviors such as smoking, in which it is now clear that any consumption is a health risk, there is no evidence that low amounts of alcohol consumption are harmful. On the contrary, there is some evidence of a health benefit at low levels, and guidance from doctors, public health, and governments vary and change over time. Currently, according to the Dietary Guidelines for Americans 2015–2020, moderate alcohol consumption is considered up to 1 drink per day for women and up to 2 drinks per day for men.[3] Therefore, the absence of a "black and white" message makes the management of alcohol problems (and not all people with alcohol problems are addicted to alcohol) very difficult.

Normal and accepted alcohol consumption varies widely in different cultures, as does the view of the cause of alcohol excess and alcohol addiction. These views range from psychosocial models of alcoholism (attributing alcoholism to factors such as upbringing or learned behaviors) to biological models, including genetic models and models of altered neurotransmitter (the chemical substance that sends messages) patterns in the brain.

The need for new drug therapies for the treatment of alcoholism

A number of medications exist that work on key proteins of the brain (receptors) and alter their activity; these medications might help some patients with alcohol addiction. However, no drug treatment for alcoholism has been shown to be effective. One drug, though, has shown promise. Baclofen is a drug given by mouth for the treatment of spasticity in cases of multiple sclerosis (a disease of the brain and spinal cord), other spinal cord diseases, and spinal cord injury; it is also prescribed off-label for alcohol use disorders. "Off-label" means that, although baclofen has not been approved as a treatment for alcohol use disorder by government regulating bodies such as the U.S. Food and Drug Administration, it can be prescribed as such.

Baclofen activates a neurotransmitter in the brain, the GABA-B receptor. The GABA-B receptor is an important part of the system that regulates the activity of the brain to prevent too-high or too-low activation. When the GABA-B receptor is activated, it decreases brain activity in various parts of the brain (inhibition). GABA receptors (GABA-A and GABA-B) are the main inhibitory receptors, and the GABA-B receptor plays a role in a number of conditions and diseases. These conditions range from movement disorders (special forms of parkinsonism), certain types of epileptic seizures (absence seizures), and certain types of headache to spasticity (for example, in multiple sclerosis or hemiplegia or tetraplegia [types of paralysis], when sometimes baclofen at relatively high doses has to be infused directly into the fluid surrounding the brain). GABA-B receptors also exist in the peripheral (non-central) nervous system and have been implicated in gastro-oesophageal reflux disease (GERD, or heartburn), chronic hiccups, and cough.

When baclofen was developed in the 1960s as part of a program to develop new anti-epileptic (anti-seizure) medications, the discovery of its role in muscle spasms led the drug company, Ciba (Basel), to invest its research and marketing resources for this use. Other uses were not actively pursued and because baclofen is inexpensive to produce and no patent for it is in force anymore, drug companies have limited interest in doing rigorous and expensive research to find or prove further indications for its use (such as re-purposing the medication for treatment of alcohol use disorders). This is why drug companies have not conducted exhaustive, large-scale studies on baclofen for the treatment of alcohol use disorder.

The baclofen controversy

To help patients worldwide with alcohol problems (who are desperate for any kind of help), a number of enthusiastic and well-regarded researchers and doctors were and are looking for medication options that might be effective in the treatment of alcohol use disorder. Baclofen has shown promise in this regard. However, the use of baclofen in the treatment of alcohol addiction is controversial. Some doctors see it as a replacement for one addiction with another (although baclofen has not been shown to be addictive); others feel that it can reduce or completely stop compulsive alcohol consumption, thereby limiting alcohol-related damage to the individual, his or her family, and society.

There is an extremely vocal and polarized debate, particularly in France, where one of the strongest baclofen advocates, Olivier Ameisen, MD, a cardiologist, lived.

Dr. Ameisen became addicted to alcohol and, desperate for any help and triggered by the positive animal research results he found, he tried baclofen on himself and describes becoming "indifferent" to alcohol through this medication. He went from consuming vast amounts of vodka to drinking only when he socialized.

Dr. Ameisen, who died of a heart attack in July 2013, wrote a book about his experiences, published in France as *Le Dernier Verre* (*The Last Glass* in English) in 2008 and in 2009 as *The End of My Addiction* in English.[4] The book received considerable attention worldwide among people with alcoholism, their families, and the doctors who treat them. Since then, large groups of patients and doctors have been advocating for its wider use, but some general practitioners and even specialists find baclofen difficult to use.

Currently, baclofen is not approved by the U.S. Food and Drug Administration for use in the treatment of alcohol use disorder, but some doctors in the United States and elsewhere (particularly in France) are prescribing it off-label for this purpose. In France, there is a government temporary recommendation for its use. Many people with alcoholism in the United States who could not get a prescription for baclofen from their doctor have turned to Internet forums to share ideas such as how to get the drug. Many of them, desperate for hope, purchase the drug from overseas pharmacies without a prescription or the supervision of a doctor; a risky practice but one many feel is worth it.

One such site is theendofmyaddiction.org, where people from all over the world share their experiences and levels of success with getting and staying sober by procuring and taking baclofen. They also share the names of doctors in the United States and Europe who are willing to prescribe baclofen off-label.

References

1. Alcohol-Related Hospital Statistics Scotland 2015/16. October 25, 2016. Available at: https://www.isdscotland.org/Health-Topics/Drugs-and-Alcohol-Misuse/Publications/2016-10-25/2016-10-25-ARHS-Report.pdf. Accessed December 29, 2016.
2. WHO Fact Sheet. Alcohol. Updated January 2015. Available at: http://www.who.int/mediacentre/factsheets/fs349/en/. Accessed November 26, 2016.
3. Appendix 9, Dietary Guidelines for Americans 2015-2020, 8th Edition. Available at: https://health.gov/dietaryguidelines/2015/guidelines/appendix-9/. Accessed December 29, 2016.
4. Ameisen O. *Le Dernier Verre.* Farrar Straus Giroux. 2008, Piatkus Press. In English, *The End of My Addiction,* 2009, New York, NY: Sarah Crichton Books.
5. de Beaurepaire R. The use of very high doses of baclofen in the treatment of alcohol dependence: a case series. *Front Psychiatry.* 2014;5:143.

About the Authors

In this book, a number of enthusiastic and internationally regarded doctors, who have all prescribed baclofen for years in the treatment of alcohol addiction, report their experiences and views and discuss the results of studies. Whether you are a patient, family member, or doctor, this book will help you understand some of the background for baclofen's use, the evidence available at present, and whether it might be a viable option for the treatment of alcoholism or alcohol withdrawal syndrome in your life or practice.

This book is also meant to spark further study of baclofen and exploration of what its role might be in society when so many people report being cured of their alcoholism through its use yet so much remains to be proven.

Following is a list of this book's lead authors, a description of their credentials, and a summary of the topics that you can expect to read about in their respective chapters.

Professor Jonathan Chick, MD, MA, MBChB, MPhil, DSc, is an experienced addiction psychiatrist who has a sound scientific background and works in Scotland, where there is a particularly widespread problem with alcohol use disorder. In Chapter 1, Dr. Chick emphasizes that such current options as talk therapy and drug treatment are not very effective in the treatment of alcohol use disorder and introduces the concept of harm reduction. Harm reduction, the concept of drinking less, which causes less damage to the person's health and the environment, has been discussed in other areas of addiction such as smoking but is relatively new in the field of alcohol use disorders.

Dr. Chick addresses the issue of the appropriate and effective dosing of baclofen, which is under constant discussion and is a source of frustration with its use. Because baclofen behaves differently in different people, doctors try to find the most effective dose for each person without causing sometimes-intolerable side effects. In general, doctors in the United Kingdom are adopting a lower highest dose compared with doctors in France, a difference due to the French experts' more biological understanding of addiction, which suggests a more biological approach to treatment.

In particular, Dr. Chick warns that doctors and patients must pay close attention to the side effects of baclofen, which (although usually mild and transient) can be severe and disabling. It is important for the treating doctors and their patients to be aware of these side effects so they can adjust the dose rapidly and to prevent any serious problems. These side effects include tiredness and mental issues (memory problems, issues with concentration, and temporary psychotic episodes). He states that baclofen is effective for some (but not all) patients, with continued questions relating to the ideal dosing regimen.

Renaud de Beaurepaire, MD, is a psychiatrist in Paris, France, where as much as 300 mg a day of baclofen has an official government license ("temporary recommendation for use"), but this is within significant procedural constraints that are currently being addressed. He has long experience with prescribing baclofen for the treatment of alcohol use disorders, and his experience has contributed significantly to the understanding of the use of this medication in alcohol addiction.

In Chapter 2, Dr. de Beaurepaire gives a short introduction on transmitters in the nervous system (neurotransmitters) and the history of the discovery of their effects in alcohol addiction. He talks about dosing, which is an important and ongoing issue. Given the highly variable amount of alcohol that patients with alcohol addiction consume and the possible differences of handling the drug in their body and in their brain, dosing of baclofen is still under intense study. For example, Dr. Ameisen, the French cardiologist introduced previously, used up to 270 mg of baclofen a day, a dosage also used in some prospective studies of individually adjusted doses.[4,5] A prospective study is one that follows a group of similar patients with certain differences over time to determine how the differences affect rates of a particular outcome.

However, most of the trials with more rigorous methodology used lower doses of baclofen. In scientific terms, methods have been used to avoid any bias from patients or researchers knowing the treatment type used. The strictest method to prove beyond a doubt that a treatment is better than another (or better than no treatment) is to compare the treatments with one another in a group of patients who are assigned their treatment by chance (in a random fashion). This is done with a placebo treatment using a non-active substance such as milk sugar and without the patient, doctor, or researcher knowing to which treatment the patient has been assigned.

This setup of a randomized, placebo-controlled, double-blind trial is expensive because of the number of people involved in the production of the drug (for example, imagine the work of putting the active drug and the placebo into similar-looking capsules labeled with identifiers only at a quantity sufficient to last for the duration of the trial), the process of the randomization (assignment of a batch of so labeled medication to 1 patient), and the rigorous documentation and controls necessary for such a trial. Such a strict methodology does not allow individualization of doses.

However, in the studies and experiences, more-highly tailored doses are used and often changed in frequent communication between the treating doctor and the patient. In communicating, doctors and patients may talk about effects such as degree of craving and the side effects of the treatment, experiences, and previous, as well as sometimes concurrent, alcohol consumption.

The experience gained through these studies, although perhaps not very rigorously obtained, cannot be denied. Dr. de Beaurepaire refers to several Internet sites, particularly in France, where information is available in forums and blogs with people sharing their experiences. Some of these sites are maintained by and for doctors, patients, or both; although the information must be interpreted with caution, these sites are useful for information exchange and for giving support and hope to people with alcohol use disorder.

Although somewhat beyond the scope of this book, Dr. de Beaurepaire mentions the use of baclofen in other addictions and the abuse of other substances such as cocaine, opiates, smoking, solvent inhalation (huffing), and binge-eating disorders. He also gives practical advice with regard to dose adjustment, which includes a proposed dosing table with a slow increase in dose being vital.

Good communication and collaboration between the doctor and the patient throughout the treatment cannot be overemphasized; therefore, I was particularly interested in Dr. de Beaurepaire's list of 10 things that must be explained to patients before prescription of baclofen, including the importance of not stopping baclofen abruptly.

Dosing adjustments are necessary because different patients have different needs; some might continue to actively drink and want to use baclofen for harm reduction; and the amount of medication varies among patients and changes over time. Dr. de Beaurepaire estimates that less than one quarter of patients need doses over 300 mg a day and feels that the treatment is most successful in highly motivated patients with supportive families.

Antonio Mirijello, MD, is part of the research group that has provided some of the most rigorous trials, with a randomized, placebo-controlled, double-blind design (described earlier) on baclofen use in patients with alcohol use disorder, in particular in patients with alcoholic liver disease. In Chapter 3,

Dr. Mirijello and colleagues also talk about the different goals, including abstinence, drinking less (harm reduction), and not going back to drinking. They also describe the importance of the GABA-B receptor in the control of drinking, reinforcement, craving, and withdrawal and outline various types of animal models for experiments to study alcohol consumption.

The authors then outline the human studies performed by their group, initially short-term and low-dose and then further randomized, controlled trials in patients with cirrhosis (scarring) of the liver with the studied endpoints (the outcomes that the researchers have set out to measure, compare, and report) of daily drinking, drink-free days, and time to relapse. They also report on an analysis of stress hormones in an open-label trial. Their work on baclofen is mentioned in guidelines from both the European Association for the Study of the Liver and the American Association for the Study of Liver Diseases.

However, not all studies show a benefit of baclofen in alcohol use disorder. In particular, a trial from the United States that treated non-hospitalized patients with a counseling intervention with the addition of baclofen or placebo and a trial from the Netherlands in which hospitalized patients were treated with intensive talk therapies. Both studies reported high rates of success in both the placebo and the baclofen groups, with no statistical difference between them, including with high-dose baclofen treatment.

The researchers believe that baclofen can help some types of patients, perhaps especially those who have certain types of craving for alcohol (relief and obsessive craving), that baclofen can be useful for the treatment of different phases of alcohol use disorder, including relapse prevention, and that it is also useful in the treatment of alcohol withdrawal syndrome.

Mehdi Farokhnia, MD, is a mental health scientist who works at the National Institutes of Health in the United States and also collaborates with the same group of researchers discussed above. In Chapter 4, these researchers report on baclofen use in alcohol withdrawal syndrome, which is a combination of severe symptoms after abrupt stoppage or rapid reduction of alcohol intake. This syndrome is experienced by many alcohol-dependent patients during the course of their disease, and the symptoms can become worse over the years, a phenomenon called "kindling."

Alcohol withdrawal symptoms can cause major distress, limit the ability of the affected person to stop drinking, and cause significant illness, complicate hospitalizations, and cause death. Symptoms typically start 6 to 24 hours after the last drink and may be mild. However, severe complications can occur as long as 72 hours after the last alcoholic drink, and life-threatening seizures and delirium tremens can result. Dr. Farokhnia and colleagues outline the role of the GABA-B receptor in the disease process of alcohol withdrawal syndrome.

During the management of the syndrome, it is important for patients to have a helpful (therapeutic) experience so that they become motivated to remain abstinent as a long-term goal. This is particularly important because if patients relapse, the alcohol withdrawal symptoms are likely to worsen, with more difficult short-term management and, likely, more treatment-resistant addiction. Many patients say that they feel stigmatized and not understood by the medical profession in this traumatic situation, which can become a medical emergency. If their encounter with the medical profession in this situation is not therapeutic, patients naturally resist engaging with difficult treatment and follow up and may return to drinking.

Medical treatment depends on the severity of the symptoms, but benzodiazepine drugs (also called tranquilizers), which increase the activity of the inhibitory GABA-A receptor, are currently the standard treatment. A number of drugs acting on this system (the GABAergic system) have been studied in alcohol withdrawal syndrome, including baclofen, and the authors begin their discussion by summarizing the results of relevant studies in animals.

Initial human experience with baclofen started with case studies of groups of patients that suggested that baclofen could be used in the treatment of alcohol withdrawal syndrome. In addition, a randomized trial comparing baclofen with the drug diazepam showed similar success in patients with uncomplicated alcohol withdrawal syndrome (absence seizures or delirium tremens, for example). A double-blind, placebo-controlled trial from 2011 studied whether the addition of baclofen to benzodiazepines (the drug lorazepam was used) was of benefit in the treatment of alcohol withdrawal syndrome. They found that patients taking baclofen were less likely to require high doses of lorazepam.

The authors believe that the future possibly lies in using tailored doses of the 2 drugs given, dependent on specific symptoms triggering the use of 1 or the other drug, thereby preventing potential dangerously high doses of benzodiazepines. It is predicted that benzodiazepines will still be in use in the future because, currently, they are the only drugs known to prevent complications of alcohol withdrawal syndrome.

However, for adherence of patients with the future treatment regimen, to decrease cravings, and to prevent relapse, there is an advantage to introducing another drug in alcohol withdrawal syndrome. The drug can then also be used in relapse prevention. In particular, the anti-anxiety effect of baclofen will likely be of benefit in the treatment of alcohol withdrawal syndrome.

Philippe Jaury, MD, works as an academic family doctor in France. In Chapter 5, Dr. Jaury discusses the side effects of baclofen and how to manage them. This important chapter reminds us that any substance that has an effect on the brain can also have sometimes-unpredictable side effects. Some of these effects are directly related to its primary action and can be similar to those of drinking too much alcohol, such as sleepiness or urinary incontinence. In my experience, some of these side effects have been seen mainly in patients in whom alcohol produced similar effects.

Reassuringly, baclofen is usually well tolerated, and most side effects are mild and improve and then disappear over time. Because baclofen has been known for more than half a century, the side effects are well known, and they can be reduced with adjustment of the dose after discussion between the patient and the treating doctor. Ways of minimizing the risk of side effects include, in particular, a slow increase in the dose.

When side effects occur, treatment must be tailored to the severity of the side effects and the motivation of the patient. Sometimes, continuation of treatment with slower-than-planned increases is indicated, but sometimes the medication must be stopped. The most common side effect, sleepiness, can often be dealt with by timing the dosing of the medication. Some side effects occur mainly when patients use alcohol while taking the medication. In particular, in people who are used to drinking very large volumes of alcohol, both the treating doctor and the patient need to be aware that some time is needed for them to find the best dose that controls the symptoms in the patient.

In addition, while the dose of baclofen is being adjusted (which has similar effects to alcohol on sleep and anxiety levels), sleep can be disrupted. However, although it can promote sleep, alcohol also disrupts sleep.

Common side effects with useful advice on how to deal with them are listed in this chapter. One important rule that every patient and treating doctor needs to be aware of is to never stop baclofen abruptly because it can cause significant side effects. These can be comparable to symptoms of severe alcohol withdrawal. Another key message of this chapter is that, since baclofen is a psychoactive drug, caution is important in patients with psychiatric illnesses.

Regular review by the treating doctor and collaboration with the doctor treating the psychiatric illness and the addiction problem is vital.

Although baclofen is a well-established drug, and over the decades there has been much experience with dosing from other fields of medicine, there are still important unanswered questions, and future research is necessary. Future research will be directed toward the understanding of the pharmacology (the study of what the drug does to the brain and body and what the body does to the drug) of baclofen in patients who continue to consume alcohol. This is different than in the group of patients with high alcohol consumption (for example, in comparison with patients with multiple sclerosis), and this is in part because of a different baseline of, for example, receptor activity that might predispose patients to the addiction.

There will also be changes in the receptor and in the handling of the medication through years of high alcohol consumption. From a practical point of view, learning which patients benefit from the medication and finding the right dosing regimens is important. One of the difficulties is to develop research methods and study designs for this medication, which depends heavily on tailored dosing within a very wide range among successfully treated patients.

Mathis Heydtmann, MD, the author of this introduction, is an experienced liver doctor (hepatologist) who has done research and worked in several countries in Europe and now works in the West of Scotland, where the rate of alcoholic liver disease is one of the highest in Europe.

Chapter One

Baclofen in an Outpatient Addiction Clinic in Scotland

Jonathan Chick, MD, MA, MBChB, MPhil, DSc, Consultant Psychiatrist; Medical Director, Castle Craig Hospital, Scotland; Visiting Professor, Edinburgh Napier University

Scotland is the only country in the world that has an alcoholic drink labeled with its nation's name. However, Scotch, especially the world-famous aged malt whiskies, is not the preferred beverage of the thousands who are addicted to alcohol in this country. When you consume large amounts of something, you need to buy it cheaply; our patients report consuming cheap cider and vodka in daily quantities equivalent to upwards of 7 ounces of ethyl alcohol, the principal alcohol in alcoholic beverages.[1] It is the ethyl alcohol to which they have become addicted.

Although Scotland has a higher death rate from alcohol than France, Spain, Italy, England, and most other Western European countries, fewer than 1 in 8 people dependent on alcohol receive treatment for their addiction.[2] Scotland is not exceptional; a World Health Organization survey found that, around the world, although 55% of people with major depression and 82% of people with schizophrenia get therapy, only about 8% of alcohol-dependent people receive treatment.[3]

The reasons for this treatment gap are several. It is common knowledge that people who develop addiction are slow to recognize, at least openly, their enslavement. If we depend on something, there is a fear of what will happen if it is no longer available. And, as for all addictions, there remains that rush of pleasure, however short-lived, that is hard to give up.

The need for a broader menu of treatments

It is widely believed that the available treatments for addiction are ineffective. Indeed, much scientific evidence informs this belief. This is frustrating. When we traced people who had attended and/or been admitted to hospitals for alcohol problems in 2 Scottish cities,[1] by 2 years, 1 in 6 of them had died. Most deaths were from preventable causes: liver disease, suicide, injuries, and accidents all related to alcohol. Even when a patient reaches a specialist treatment service using individual and group therapy, perhaps only 15% are helped to be abstinent or are drinking without problems at the 2-year point, which is little better than if they had only received 1 session of "advice," or talk therapy.[4]

Some people who, in a door-to-door or telephone survey, report a pattern of drinking and symptoms that suggests dependence, never get help and yet, when they are re-interviewed some years later, have recovered; about 5% to 45% of people have this pattern of drinking.[5,6] Others come into treatment and might be more severely addicted in some way, but their recovery rates are not much better than those of people who never received treatment, especially in the longer term.[7]

Which treatments have been shown to be effective? There is evidence that Alcoholics Anonymous (AA) helps many,[7] but although the exact figure is unknown, many of whom have been introduced to the AA program do not stick to it or, even if they do, relapse.

Are any treatments for alcohol use disorder effective?

The correct scientific method to assess the effectiveness of a treatment is to run a comparison with a dummy treatment (placebo). This evens out between the 2 test groups other aspects of therapy (for example, the effect of the dialog that takes place between the doctor and the patient and the attendance at the clinic, which can have a motivational effect). However, even a study conducted with a control group may give a biased result, perhaps due to the researchers' expectations or the kind of patient who has been included.

Thus, it is widely accepted that, when possible, results of all studies should be combined and analyzed together, as researchers Jonas and colleagues did for 123 distinct studies of various medications developed to prevent relapse in alcohol use disorder.[8] They found that, for every medicine tested, at least half of the patients are not helped or drop out because of side effects. And while the drug disulfiram, which results in unpleasant side effects when the user drinks alcohol, can be quite effective for some, a benefit emerges only when someone watches the person take the tablet to make sure they take it (for example, a partner, pharmacist, or employer), which is something that not all patients can implement for themselves or will comply with.

One way in which doctors rate the effectiveness of a medication is to examine how many patients need to be treated with the medication to achieve a good outcome compared with the number of those who have a good outcome with only the placebo. Jonas and colleagues found that a doctor needs to treat 12 patients with the drug acamprosate to prevent 1 extra person from relapsing than would have been achieved with placebo; for naltrexone, the number is 20. And for 1 extra person to be prevented from returning to heavy drinking who would not have achieved that on placebo (that is, not necessarily totally abstinent), the doctor would have to prescribe naltrexone to 12 patients.[8] Now, placebo pills are "effective" in many conditions, including depression, pain, and even some infectious diseases, but in day-to-day practice, doctors do not give the placebo because they are usually obliged to be honest with the patient.

So doctors continue to prescribe these medications because they are the only ones approved for alcohol use disorder. Or they prescribe something approved but ineffective. For example, antidepressants are often prescribed to problem drinkers.[9] In fact, they seldom help the depression and have been proven to have no benefit for the drinking[10,11]; indeed, the selective serotonin reuptake inhibitors (for example, Prozac), which are the most commonly prescribed antidepressants, have been shown, on average, to cause *more* drinking, especially in patients whose drinking problems began before age 25 years.[12–15]

Why baclofen?

The need for alternative treatments for alcohol problems is clear. In Scotland, we have been aware of what other chapters of this book have charted: the discovery that the GABA-B receptor had a role in alcohol dependence in animals and that the use of baclofen in animals bred to be dependent on alcohol reduced their interest in alcohol. When we read about the work of researchers Addolorato and colleagues in the liver clinic in Rome (see Chapter 3), we carefully began to try baclofen, at first only in the patients who had tried various treatment approaches but kept relapsing.

Although doctors in the United Kingdom are not authorized by the national medicines agency to prescribe baclofen for alcoholism, an individual doctor may do so if he or she has specialist knowledge and medical indemnity insurance. To help us in Scotland, the evidence was sufficient to convince some local health authorities to permit a specialist clinic to prescribe baclofen for our patients at no cost to the patient (in fact, the cost per tablet was minimal).

At first, we prescribed only to patients who had established a few days of abstinence, after medically assisted withdrawal from alcohol. This, it turned out, was not the way in which Olivier Ameisen, MD, had managed to stop drinking, as described in his article submitted in 2004 as a "single-case self-report"[16] to the scientific journal that I edited, *Alcohol and Alcoholism*. He had started to take baclofen while still consuming large amounts of alcohol and gradually found with increasing doses (eventually, very high doses) that he had lost his urge to drink alcohol and could stay abstinent.

As in Dr. Ameisen's biographical account,[16,17] we have sometimes prescribed baclofen to patients who are still drinking, with some (but not all) achieving gradual reduction of alcohol consumption. Our preference is to start the baclofen after detoxification. Dr. Ameisen graphically described his tendency to have anxiety, and we have veered toward offering baclofen to patients whose triggers to drinking include anxiety. Subsequent studies have sometimes,[18] but not always,[19] found that a tendency toward anxiety predicts a good response to baclofen treatment.

If baclofen, what dose?

In the United Kingdom, the national recommendation is that baclofen should not be prescribed above 100 mg a day. We have found that many patients maintain abstinence or much reduced drinking on doses of 30 to 90 mg a day. The peer-reviewed studies of the Addolorato group had demonstrated safety and effectiveness on up to 60 mg a day. At the time of this writing, only 1 peer-reviewed published report has shown safety and effectiveness above 100 mg a day.[20] Other case reports of higher doses have been published in peer-reviewed journals in which up to 140 mg a day was used.[21]

However, in France, many prescriptions have followed the route described by Dr. Ameisen in his self-report. The enthusiasm with which higher doses have been prescribed by French doctors has surprised some observers. Interestingly, it is known that specialists in France, compared with those of some other countries, have long tended to espouse the biological understanding of alcohol addiction rather than the "moral" perception of alcohol excess as a choice.[22] This would incline these specialists to use a chemical instead of or as well as a psychological or social approach.

Unwanted side effects that cause concern

On initiating baclofen treatment, many people feel slightly sedated or even dizzy. If the starting dose is low (for example, 5 mg 2 or 3 times a day), the sedation is not severe and tends to pass, allowing a gradual increase to a dose of, say, 30 mg to 80 mg a day. At that level, patients report that they no longer feel the urge to drink alcohol, can more easily resist temptation, and are free of unwanted sedative effects. There is an increase in unwanted sedation as the dose increases and if alcohol is consumed.[23]

While some patients report better sleep than they knew in their years of drinking, for others, a difficulty with getting to sleep emerges. There is a serious unwanted effect in some people who have taken doses higher than 100 mg a day; such doses seem to provoke the mind to overactivity and excitement so that the mind embroiders and embellishes experiences out of touch with reality, and behavior is disinhibited and out of character. This can be dangerous; one man believed that he had discovered a method of winning at online gambling and lost large sums of money, while another started talking nonstop, sleeping for only 3 hours per night and, for the first time, using an online dating service. Psychiatrists term this "psychosis of a manic type." There can also be a paranoid tinge to the perceptions so that the person feels slights where none were intended or imagines threats. These effects pass with gradual withdrawal of the baclofen, perhaps with the need for a brief prescription of an antipsychotic medication. There have been several reports of this pattern.[24]

At the time of this writing, the most recent report of a baclofen controlled trial was conducted in the Netherlands and found that patients allocated into a "high"-dose group had trouble tolerating doses above 100 mg a day.[25] (It is also of interest that this study failed to show an advantage to baclofen at either low/moderate or higher doses above the result found for the placebo group. Subjects had been recruited from 2 residential programs, one of which was 4 weeks long and applied the 12-step treatment method popularized by Alcoholics Anonymous. The other program was of 6 weeks duration and was based on cognitive behavioral therapy principles. High levels of abstinence [about 50%] were found in all groups at the 4-month point, perhaps contributing to difficulty showing any effect of baclofen.)

Older patients may notice impaired memory and concentration, which also can have serious consequences. Reduction of the dose may relieve that unwanted effect. There are also reports of extreme anxiety with distortion of thinking during sudden withdrawal from high doses of baclofen.[26]

Conclusions

With careful research, in time we will learn which people who are dependent on alcohol can safely benefit from baclofen. There will be some who cannot tolerate the side effects and some for whom it is ineffective. Some, probably severely addicted people, will find that baclofen provides an answer that they could not find in other treatments. For how long the latter group should take baclofen, and in what dose, remains to be answered. Baclofen is a substance that alters brain cell transmissions, and it should be used with care.

References
1. Gill, J, Black H, Chick J, et al. Alcohol purchasing by ill heavy drinkers; cheap alcohol is no single commodity. *Public Health.* 2015. Available at: http://dx.doi. org/10.1016/j.puhe.2015.08.013. Accessed October 10, 2016.
2. NHS Health Scotland. Assessing the availability of and need for specialist alcohol treatment services in Scotland. 2014. Available at: http://www.healthscotland.com/documents/24408.aspx. Accessed October 10, 2016.
3. Kohn R, Saxena S, Levav I, Saraceno B. The treatment gap in mental health care. *Bull World Health Organ.* 2004;82(11):858-66. Epub 2004 Dec. 14. Review.
4. Chick J, Ritson B, Connaughton J, Stewart A. Advice versus extended treatment for alcoholism: a controlled study. *Br J Addict.* 1988;83:159-70.
5. Armor DJ, Meshkoff JE. Remission among treated and untreated alcoholics. *Adv Subst Abuse.* 1983;3:239–69.
6. Roizen R, Cahalan D, Shanks P. "Spontaneous remission" among untreated problem drinkers. In: Kandel DB, ed. *Longitudinal Research on Drug Use: Empirical Findings and Methodological Issues.* Washington, DC: Hemisphere; 1978. pp. 197–221.
7. Moos RH[1], Moos BS. Sixteen-year changes and stable remission among treated and untreated individuals with alcohol use disorders. *Drug Alcohol Depend.* 2005 Dec 12;80(3):337-47.
8. Jonas DE, Amick HR, Feltner C, et al. Pharmacotherapy for adults with alcohol use disorders in outpatient settings: a systematic review and meta-analysis. *JAMA.* 2014 May 14;311(18):1889-900.

9. Foulds JA, Rouch S, Spence J, Mulder RT, Sellman JD. Prescribed psychotropic medication use in patients receiving residential addiction treatment *Alcohol.* 2016;51(5):622-23.
10. Torrens M, Fonseca F, Mateu G, Farré M. Efficacy of antidepressants in substance use disorders with and without comorbid depression. A systematic review and meta-analysis. *Drug Alcohol Depend.* 2005 Apr 4;78(1):1-22.
11. Iovieno N, Tedeschini E, Bentley KH, Evins AE, Papakostas GI. Antidepressants for major depressive disorder and dysthymic disorder in patients with comorbid alcohol use disorders: a meta-analysis of placebo-controlled randomized trials. *J Clin Psychiatry.* 2011 Aug;72(8):1144-51.
12. Pettinati HM, Volpicelli JR, Luck G, et al. Double-blind clinical trial of sertraline treatment for alcohol dependence. *J Clin Psychopharmacol.* 2001;21:143-153.
13. Charney DA, Heath LM, Zikos E, Palacios-Boix J, Gill KJ. Poorer drinking outcomes with citalopram treatment for alcohol dependence: a randomized, double-blind, placebo-controlled trial. *Alcohol Clin Exp Res.* 2015;39(9):1756-65.
14. Chick J, Aschauer H, Hornik K. Efficacy of fluvoxamine in preventing relapse in alcohol dependence: a one-year, double-blind, placebo-controlled multicentre study with analysis by typology. *Drug Alcohol Depend.* 2004;74:61-70.
15. Kranzler HR, Del Boca FK, Rounsaville BJ. Comorbid psychiatric diagnosis predicts three-year outcomes in alcoholics: a posttreatment natural history study. *J Stud Alcohol.* 1996;57:619-26.
16. Ameisen O. Complete and prolonged suppression of symptoms and consequences of alcohol-dependence using high-dose baclofen: a self-case report of a physician. *Alcohol.* 2005;40(2):147-50.
17. Ameisen O. *Le Dernier Verre* 2008. Farrar Straus Giroux (in English, *The End of My Addiction,* 2009, Piatkus Press).
18. Morley KC, Baillie A, Leung S, Addolorato G, Leggio L, Haber PS. Baclofen for the treatment of alcohol dependence and possible role of comorbid anxiety. *Alcohol.* 2014;49(6):654-60.
19. Müller CA, Geisel O, Pelz P, et al. High-dose baclofen for the treatment of alcohol dependence (BACLAD study): a randomized, placebo-controlled trial. *Eur Neuropsychopharmacol.* 2015;25(8):1167-77.
20. Addolorato G, Leggio L, Ferrulli A, et al. Dose-response effect of baclofen in reducing daily alcohol intake in alcohol dependence: secondary analysis of a randomized, double-blind, placebo-controlled trial. *Alcohol.* 2011;46:312-17.
21. Bucknam W. Suppression of symptoms of alcohol dependence and craving using high-dose baclofen. *Alcohol.* 2007;42:158-60.
22. Koski-Jännes A, Pennonen M, Simmat-Durand L. Treatment professionals' basic beliefs about alcohol use disorders: different cultural contexts. *Subst Use Misuse.* 2016;51(4):479-88.
23. Rolland B, Labreuche J, Duhamel A, et al. Baclofen for alcohol dependence: Relationships between baclofen and alcohol dosing and the occurrence of major sedation. *Eur Neuropsychopharmacol.* 2015 Oct;25(10):1631-6.
24. Geoffroy PA, Auffret M, Deheul S, et al. Baclofen-induced manic symptoms: case report and systematic review. *Psychosomatics.* 2014 Jul-Aug;55(4):326-32.
25. Beraha EM, Salemink E, Goudriaan AE, et al. Efficacy and safety of high-dose

baclofen for the treatment of alcohol dependence: A multicentre, randomised, double-blind controlled trial. *Eur Neuropsychopharmacology.* 2016.
26(12):1950-9.

26. Rolland B, Jaillette E, Carton L, et al. Assessing alcohol versus baclofen withdrawal syndrome in patients treated with baclofen for alcohol use disorder. *J
Clin Psychopharmacol.* 2014 Feb;34(1):153-6.

Chapter Two

Individual Adjustment of Baclofen Dosage to Treat Alcohol Dependence

Renaud de Beaurepaire, MD, Groupe Hospitalier Paul-Guiraud, Villejuif, France

Alcohol abuse and dependence are major public health problems, with an estimated social cost of 120 billion Euro (about $136 billion) per year in France.[1] Several medications are approved for the treatment of alcohol dependence, including acamprosate, naltrexone, nalmefene, and disulfiram, but these drugs are not very effective in the treatment of alcoholism, and alcohol dependence remains a difficult-to-treat condition.[2]

Baclofen, a drug that has been used for more than 40 years in the treatment of spasticity (a condition in which the muscles stiffen, affecting movement or speech), has shown promise in the treatment of alcohol dependence. Interest in baclofen for the treatment of alcohol-related problems goes back to studies in the 1970s, when researchers showed that rats under the influence of alcohol displayed fewer alcohol-related behaviors when given baclofen, leading the researchers to conclude that baclofen may be useful in the treatment of chronic alcoholism.[3]

Eleven years later, another group of researchers showed that baclofen reduces the use of alcohol in alcohol-preferring rats and stated that the moderation of voluntary alcohol intake could be related to a change in how the brain uses the neurotransmitter GABA (GABA reduces the activity of nerve cells) and responds to stimulation of GABA-B receptors (baclofen boosts the effects of GABA).[4]

Later, other researchers showed that baclofen prevents animals from developing a tolerance to cocaine and reduces cocaine's stimulant effects[5], and other researchers showed that baclofen reduces the consumption of cocaine in rats.[6] The ability of baclofen to reduce alcohol consumption in rats who preferred alcohol to water was confirmed by a 2002 study.[7] These animal test results linking addiction to GABA-B receptors confirmed previous human studies showing that sodium oxybate (commonly known as GHB), a stimulant of GABA-B receptors, is effective in the treatment of alcohol dependence.[8]

Sodium oxybate and baclofen both activate GABA-B receptors, but they differ in their effects on other neurotransmitters. Baclofen reduces the release of the neurotransmitter dopamine, while sodium oxybate activates it (a potential cause of sodium oxybate abuse).[9] Baclofen does not act on other neurotransmitters, while sodium oxybate acts on serotonin, norepinephrine, and opiate systems.[10] Together, these animal and human studies prompted further studies looking at the effect of baclofen on alcohol use disorder.

Individual adjustment of baclofen dosage in alcohol dependence

The first human studies evaluating the effect of baclofen in the treatment of alcohol dependence used low doses (30 to 60 mg a day). The results were con-flicting, with some studies showing that baclofen was effective[11–15] and others showing no effects.[16–18] In the meantime, several single-case reports were pub-lished[19–22] that showed that the dose of baclofen necessary for a given patient varies widely, is most often far higher than 60 mg, and that when the dose is adjusted for a particular patient, baclofen can be very effective in reducing cravings for alcohol.

One of these reports mentioned earlier in this book, from Olivier Ameisen, MD, had a major impact.[19] Ameisen was a French doctor who had a brilliant career as a cardiologist in New York but became an alcoholic and then later cured himself with a high dose of baclofen (270 mg a day). He wrote a book about his cure, *The End of My Addiction*,[23] which was an editorial success, was translated into many languages, and received a great deal of worldwide media attention. The result was that thousands of alcohol-dependent patients began seeking baclofen treatment, urging thousands of doctors reluctant to prescribe an off-label use of a drug (using it to treat conditions other than what it has been approved for) at unusual and possibly dangerous doses.

Most doctors declined to prescribe it but, facing their patients' distress, many have prescribed it for compassionate use (prescribing an unapproved drug for seriously ill patients who have no other effective treatment options). It rapidly became obvious to these doctors that tailored baclofen treatment had a high and never-before-achieved effectiveness in the treatment of alcohol use disorder.

A series of prospective studies was published involving a large number of patients who were monitored over long periods of time. These studies independently reported similar results: when baclofen was individually adjusted, with no assigned upper limit of the dose, about 50% of patients became effortlessly indifferent to alcohol and stopped drinking, while 20% to 30% appeared to be unable to stop drinking completely but did reduce their drinking considerably.[24–28]

Another remarkable result was that the beneficial effects of baclofen were long lasting, with one study showing that, 2 years after beginning treatment, 62% of patients still did not drink or drank moderately.[28] These results are different from those obtained with approved treatments, which have never shown any effectiveness over the long term.

The effectiveness of baclofen was recently confirmed in 2 randomized, controlled, double-blind studies (studies in which patients were randomly given baclofen or placebo [inactive drug], but neither they nor the researchers knew which they had been given), the BACLAD study[29] and the Bacloville study.[30] In these 2 studies, the treatment dose was individually adjusted, and the maximum allowable dose of baclofen was high (270 mg a day in the BACLAD study and 300 mg a day in the Bacloville study).

In the BACLAD study, 68.2% of the baclofen-treated patients did not drink during the adjusted dose period (3 months) versus 28.8% in the placebo group. In the Bacloville study, which lasted 1 year, 56.8% of the patients did not drink at all or only moderately (within a normal range, according to World Health Organization criteria) at the end of the study versus 36.5% in the placebo group.

The statistical difference between baclofen and placebo was highly significant in both studies. The average dose of baclofen was 180 mg a day in the BACLAD study and 160 mg a day in the Bacloville study (this means that about half of the patients needed more than these doses to stop craving alcohol).

Interestingly, the results of 2 other randomized, controlled, double-blind studies were also recently released, the Alpadir study[31] and the Dutch study,[32] in which low maximal (ceiling) doses were used (180 mg a day in the Alpadir study and 150 mg a day in the Dutch study). The results of these studies were negative, or showed that baclofen was not more effective than placebo. These negative results are easy to understand because ceiling doses of 150 and 180 mg a day are clearly not enough (as mentioned previously, about half of the patients need more than these doses). The negative results of the Alpadir and Dutch studies confirm that baclofen treatment must be individually adjusted with a high (or no assigned) upper limit of the dose.

In a personal study, using no assigned upper limit of dose, I showed that 24% of the patients needed doses equal to or higher than 300 mg a day to stop drinking.[33] Similarly, in the Bacloville study, 25% of the patients needed doses higher than 242 mg a day.

Taken together, the results of randomized and nonrandomized studies converge to show that the dose response to baclofen is highly variable, with some patients needing small doses and others needing high or very high doses. The reasons for these differences are unknown. An important relationship has been reported between the amount of alcohol consumed before treatment and the required dose of baclofen,[28] but many other factors are likely involved, including an important difference in how the drug works in different people.[34] The influence of genetic, or hereditary, factors is currently under investigation in France.

Individually adjusted baclofen in conditions other than alcohol dependence

Baclofen has been used in the treatment of many conditions other than alcohol dependence. There also, the question of individual dose adjustment appears to be critical. The most classic example of a need for individual baclofen adjustment is its use for the first time in neurological disorders causing spasticity. Neurologists (doctors who treat diseases of the brain, spinal cord, and nerves) have long reported that the effective dose of baclofen in the treatment of spasticity often goes far beyond the maximum recommended dose (about 80 mg a day, depending on the country), commonly reaching 300 mg a day, even in children.[35] It was noted[35] that high doses of baclofen did not spur patients to stop taking it due to unwanted side effects.

Baclofen has also been tried as a treatment for cocaine dependence. Three studies, all using low doses of baclofen (60 mg a day) have been published. The first two reported positive results[36,37] (meaning that baclofen was shown to be effective), while the third, a randomized, controlled, double-blind trial, reported that baclofen was not effective in the treatment of cocaine addiction.[38] In this latter study, the researchers acknowledged that trials using doses higher than 60 mg were warranted. A number of small studies using low doses have also been conducted in other types of substance abuse, including opiate withdrawal,[39] alcohol withdrawal,[40–42] cigarette smoking,[43] and solvent inhalation (often called "huffing").[44]

Although these studies reported that baclofen was effective, most raised serious concerns about the design of the study and how it could have influenced the results; for example, a meta-analysis concluded that baclofen cannot be recommended for the treatment of alcohol withdrawal.[45] These studies need to be redone using more people and higher doses of baclofen.

The effects of baclofen in eating disorders also illustrate the need for a tailored dose. Animal studies have shown that baclofen reduces binge fat consumption[46,47] and sugar consumption,[48,49] opening the way for human studies. Two clinical studies have examined the effects of low-dose baclofen (60 mg a day) in patients with binge-eating disorder.[50,51] The results showed that baclofen was, overall, effective, but only a minority of patients became completely free of binge eating in these studies.

Given that individually adjusted baclofen is presumably more effective than low doses in the treatment of alcohol dependence, a number of French doctors started prescribing individually adjusted off-label baclofen in binge-eating disorder and bulimia nervosa (a pattern of binging and vomiting). The results appear to be globally similar to those seen in alcohol use disorder (about 50% of patients were completely free of binge episodes, 20% were in partial remission, and 30% found that the treatment did not work for them). These results are still unpublished (submitted) except a short series of clinical cases.[52]

Besides alcohol and eating disorders, baclofen has also shown to be effective in several stomach disorders such as hiccups,[53] rumination (regurgitation of food), aerophagia (swallowing of air), and supragastric belching (belching of air from above the stomach),[54,55] but only low doses have been used in the treatment of these conditions. French prescribers also often successfully use individually adjusted off-label baclofen in the treatment of behavioral disturbances and self-mutilation (cutting) in patients with various conditions, including borderline personality disorder and mental retardation. The use of baclofen in patients with mental retardation who self-mutilate has been reported to be effective.[56]

Patient interactions and Internet baclofen sites

Following the release of Dr. Ameisen's book in France, several doctors who successfully treated patients created Internet sites, forums, and blogs, providing full information in French about baclofen in alcohol dependence and were dedicated to the sharing of experiences between baclofen users and prescribers. The site AUBES (baclofene.fr/portal.php) was created in 2009 by both doctors and patients; the site Baclofène (baclofene.org) was created in 2011 by and for patients; and the site RESAB (http://resab.fr) was created in 2012 by and for doctors (it has now become a site for the medical education of doctors who wish to prescribe baclofen).

AUBES, Baclofène, and RESAB are primarily nonprofit associations with a goal of promoting knowledge about the practice of prescribing baclofen for the treatment of alcohol use disorder. Members of these associations have been active with the media and government authorities. Articles and editorials were published, conferences were organized, a manifesto was launched, several books written by patients were published, and meetings with French Health Ministry representatives were requested. However, the Internet sites have been the most useful tools.

The Baclofène Internet site has more than 10,000 active members, which means that more than 10,000 patients say that they have been taking baclofen for their alcohol use disorder, and most of the time, these patients report that baclofen has been very useful. The site has more than 3,000 visitors per day. Several hundreds of thousands of between-patient discussions have taken place in the forum since its creation. Most of the discussions deal with baclofen adjustment, states of craving and side effects.

When thousands of people publicly acknowledge that they have been cured by a given medication, is it really necessary to conduct long, complex, and costly clinical trials with an uncertain outcome? Such patient activism has irritated many people, and some have denounced the "French craze for baclofen."[53] But what if there were no craze, only good medicine?

Besides the spread of information about baclofen treatment of alcoholism in the general public, the Internet groups have had some success with French health authorities. Clearly under the pressure of patient groups, the French Health Safety Agency released in March 2014 a "temporary recommendation for use" (TRU) allowing the prescription of baclofen of up to 300 mg a day for the treatment of alcohol dependence. The TRU was followed in

June 2014 by a Health Ministry statement that baclofen for the treatment of alcohol dependence, up to 300 mg a day, would be given free of charge.

The TRU was a great victory for the patient groups because it was official recognition of the advantages of baclofen in the treatment of alcohol dependence and because it acknowledged that high doses may be necessary even though the TRU rapidly proved to be difficult for doctors to use in daily practice because of complex procedural constraints.[54] The TRU is currently being changed to address these concerns.

Baclofen prescription and dose adjustment

Baclofen reduces cravings, and all baclofen-treated patients should benefit from this effect. However, in practice, the prescription of baclofen is not simple. As mentioned earlier, the effective dose of baclofen can vary greatly from one patient to another, ranging from a few tens to several hundred milligrams, and the dose must be individually tailored. When a patient is seen for the first time, the doctor has no way of knowing the effective dose.

Baclofen also produces many side effects (see Chapter 5), and the side effects are also highly variable and unpredictable from one patient to another. Some patients tolerate very high doses of baclofen with no noticeable side effects, while others do not tolerate even a single tablet. Side effects can occur at any time and at any dose. It is generally accepted (though not clearly shown) that baclofen dosages must be increased very slowly to minimize side effects.

The principle of baclofen prescription is to slowly increase the dose until the patient has no more craving for alcohol, or, in Dr. Ameisen's words, until the patient becomes "indifferent" to alcohol.

When a doctor sees a patient for the first time, he or she must explain all these things thoroughly to the patient: the effective dose is not known for a given patient; the doses are slowly increased until cravings go away; the dose increase is very often slowed or prevented due to side effects; and the challenge is to reach the effective dose despite the side effects. The patient must understand this challenge and be personally involved in the progression of the treatment. The patient's cooperation with the doctor is fundamental for baclofen treatment. Without this relationship, the patient may quickly stop the treatment, arguing that he or she does not tolerate the side effects, thus losing the opportunity to be cured of alcoholism.

Internet forums are often of great help to patients, allowing them to note that they are not the only ones to have difficulties with side effects and to share with others their personal experiences and questions.

10 things that must be discussed with a patient before prescription

Before baclofen is prescribed, several precautions must be taken to minimize the risk of certain side effects or medical accidents. Following are 10 items that need to be discussed with a patient before treatment begins:

1) Baclofen has sedative effects. Sedative effects are the most common side effect of baclofen; they are most often tolerable but are sometimes intense, with sleepiness and the risk of falling asleep abruptly. Driving a car or using potentially dangerous tools (for example, an electric saw) is forbidden during the first weeks of treatment until patients learn how the sedation affects them. Patients must be informed that sedation is often accompanied by instability or balance problems and that they must plan their daily life with these symptoms in mind. Daytime sleepiness is also often associated with an inability to sleep at night.

2) Doctors must be cautious when prescribing baclofen to patients with breathing and heart problems. Baclofen may slow breathing, can worsen sleep apnea (a condition featuring frequent pauses in breathing during sleep), and can decrease blood pressure and heart rate. Reduced breathing and circulation can lead to a lack of oxygen, increasing the risk of a cardiac event. In the case of sleep apnea, the patient must be treated with a positive airway pressure mask.

   Rates of problems related to breathing and the heart increase with age, and doctors must be very cautious when using baclofen in elderly patients. Baclofen cannot be used in patients with a history of stroke and, in general, is not recommended for those who are in poor physical health. However, there is no reason that people older than 70 years should not benefit from baclofen if they are in good physical health.

3) Baclofen can promote seizures in people with a history of epilepsy and in those with no history of seizures. In the first case, epilepsy drug treatment may need to be increased. Otherwise, the patient must be aware that epilepsy is a possibility due to the interaction of baclofen and alcohol; one

case was reported of new-onset seizures in a patient with no history of epilepsy who was taking baclofen and abusing alcohol at the same time.[59]

4) Baclofen has caused cases of mania and depression. However, this is a complex issue. Baclofen can certainly trigger mania in patients with bipolar disorder. Baclofen prescribers must therefore look for a history of bipolarity in patients, inform them about the risks of relapse, possibly increase the dose of mood stabilizers or add an extra mood stabilizer, and, above all, vigilantly monitor patients with frequent visits and explanations about symptoms of a relapse. One study, however, reported the probable occurrence of new-onset mania in a patient with no history of bipolarity,[60] indicating that doctors must be alert to the warning signs of mania in all patients.

It can be difficult to monitor the occurrence of hypomania, or low-level mania. Baclofen triggered hypomanic episodes in about 7% of the patients in a 2012 study.[28] In hypomania, patients tend to feel very well, are happy and active, sleep less than usual, and are more effective in their work. In most cases, hypomania is benign; is well tolerated by patients, relatives, and coworkers; and does not precede mania, providing no reason to decrease baclofen treatment or slow the dose increase.

On the other hand, depression is not uncommon in patients taking baclofen. However, alcohol dependence itself is associated with depression in about 50% of cases, according to a 2000 study,[61] so it is generally difficult to blame baclofen when a baclofen-treated patient becomes depressed. Nevertheless, baclofen may cause depression on its own and, in any event, the baclofen dose must be decreased when a patient becomes depressed during treatment, all the more so if the patient has suicidal thoughts. The patient must be informed that he or she has to decrease the dose of baclofen in the case of suicidal thoughts. The use of antidepressants is often helpful for the treatment of depression during baclofen treatment.

5) It is essential to ask for a creatinine blood test when starting baclofen. Because baclofen is mostly excreted from the body by the kidneys, it builds up in patients with kidney failure, rapidly causing symptoms of drug accumulation and confusion.

6) Patients must be aware that baclofen can cause a wide range of sometimes very intense sensations, most likely due to high concentrations of GABA-B receptors on sensory pathways (for example, tinnitus [ringing or whistling in the ears]; pain; sensations of electric shocks; changes in

smell, vision, and taste; and sometimes, hallucinations and vivid night-mares). These feelings and sensory effects can be extremely upsetting for the patient, and the doctor must explain that they are benign, will disap-pear when the baclofen dosage is decreased, and do not call for a change to the prescription.

7) Patients with Parkinson's disease must be treated carefully because baclofen worsens the side effects of levodopa (the gold-standard drug for the treatment of Parkinson's disease, levodopa is converted to dopamine in the brain), possibly causing hallucinations, delusions, and confusion. In addition, baclofen reduces transmission of the neurotransmitter dopa-mine (the neurotransmitter that is lacking in the brains of patients with Parkinson's disease), which may worsen Parkinson's symptoms.

8) Patients should be informed that baclofen treatment must not be abruptly stopped. Abrupt baclofen stoppage, mostly when high doses are taken, can cause a series of symptoms that, interestingly, resemble abrupt alco-hol stoppage in heavy drinkers: confusion, hallucinations, delusions, and seizures. This raises the idea that baclofen may be in some way a substi-tute for alcohol.

9) A series of questions also need to be asked of patients:
   • Do they have a history of peptic ulcer (because baclofen can trigger them)?
   • Do they have urinary incontinence, which is worsened by baclofen?
   • Are they taking medications that may interact with baclofen (because baclofen is rapidly excreted by the kidneys, these interactions are very few)?
   • Do they react badly to the inactive ingredients in tablets (for example, gluten in some generic forms)?

   Drug information often emphasizes that prescribers should be par-ticularly cautious in prescribing baclofen to patients with psychosis, diabetes, liver disease, or porphyria (a group of rare diseases in which porphyrin pigments build up in the body). In my experience, these con-ditions should not limit the use of baclofen. In particular, patients with schizophrenia, a severe mental illness that features psychosis, can clearly benefit from baclofen. Several studies have shown that baclofen is well tolerated in patients with cirrhosis (scarring of the liver due to alcohol abuse or disease),[13] and baclofen is obviously less toxic (if it is toxic at all) than alcohol on liver cells.

10) Women of childbearing age raise a genuine ethical problem when it comes to baclofen treatment for alcoholism. Alcohol dependence during pregnancy is a serious issue. In France, 6,000 children are born every year with deformities related to their mother's alcoholism. Drug information advises against the use of baclofen during pregnancy. However, no case of deformity or other kind of birth defect has ever been reported after the use of baclofen during pregnancy (except baclofen withdrawal symptoms in the newborn). The benefit/risk ratio should therefore favor baclofen. However, unfortunately, most baclofen prescribers remain reluctant to prescribe baclofen to alcohol-dependent women who are pregnant or at risk for becoming pregnant.

When these 10 items are fully investigated and discussed with patients before starting treatment, management of baclofen treatment is much less complicated. The patients feel involved in the treatment after the discussion that sets up the doctor-patient commitment to treatment. The prescribing doctor must then thoroughly explain to the patient and his or her family the management of the treatment.

Dosage increases must occur with regularity. Many side effects occur because patients do not strictly follow the dose increase pattern. However, there is no clearly established dose increase pattern. Most doctors in France propose an increase of 10 mg every 3 days, but many propose a slower increase (for example, 10 mg every 5 or 7 days). Usually, doses are given 3 times daily (morning, noon, and evening), but some doctors prefer doses to be taken 5 times daily, or every 2 hours during the waking hours.

The best way to prescribe baclofen is to target the period of craving: baclofen must be given during the hour that precedes the occurrence of craving. For instance, in those who drink only in the evening, baclofen should be given only in the evening, during the hour that usually precedes the start of drinking.

Baclofen has a half-life of about 4 hours, which means that half of the medication is still active in the body after 4 hours. However, the way baclofen works in the brain is not fully understood. Patients must be involved in their treatment; they have to continue learning how to manage and change doses according to the occurrence of side effects, the time of the day they usually drink alcohol, and the effect of the treatment on their daily activities.

When a difficult-to-tolerate side effect occurs, dose increases should slow for a while, or the dosage should be reduced by 1 or 2 tablets; a few days later, when the side effect has disappeared or is bearable, the dose can be increased again more slowly (for example, using half tablets with increases every week or every 2 weeks). The principle is to progressively overcome the barrier of side effects and increase the dose until the craving for alcohol is gone or at least greatly reduced.

The decrease or stoppage of craving occurs in almost all patients who are able to increase the dosage to one that is effective for them. However, this does not mean that all patients stop drinking. The craving-reducing effect may not be strong enough, or the patients may be too strongly attached to their drinking habits. Nevertheless, in general, when the dose that decreases or stops cravings is reached, most patients greatly reduce the amount of alcohol they drink.

Conclusions and future directions

Baclofen is a powerful alcohol-craving reducer, but the management of baclofen treatment in alcohol-related disorders is often difficult. Given that the effective dose varies widely from one patient to another, the dose must be individually tailored; the goal of the treatment is to increase the dose until the patient no longer craves alcohol. However, baclofen can have many side effects that are often difficult to tolerate and are potentially dangerous; thus, the dose increase is often reduced or slowed by unbearable side effects.

Therefore, the second goal of the treatment is the doctor-patient relationship in which the patient becomes personally involved, with the support of the doctor, in monitoring the treatment. This is essential when the side effects are intense and high doses must be reached for craving suppression. The need for very high doses to stop cravings is not unusual.

I have previously mentioned the Bacloville study, in which 25% of the patients needed doses higher than 242 mg a day.[30] I also mentioned a personal study that showed that 24% of baclofen-treated alcohol-dependent patients needed doses equal to or greater than 300 mg a day.[33] In this study, the patients reaching such doses were, in general, highly motivated to stop alcohol cravings. Their involvement in the management of the treatment (often with the family's involvement) proved to be essential to the success of the treatment. Several of these patients also used the support of Internet forums.

Future directions are many. We need to find out why the necessary dosage of baclofen varies so much from patient to patient. I have seen differences in the ways different patients' bodies use baclofen, and I have mentioned possible genetic variations. I have also reported that there is a significant relationship between the amount of alcohol consumed before treatment and the required dose of baclofen; this raises the possibility of differences in how much the brain has changed as a result of chronic alcohol abuse and the intensity of the patient's attachment to alcohol. Imaging studies (for example, magnetic resonance imaging [MRI] or computed tomography [CT]) looking at brain activities in baclofen-treated alcohol-dependent patients are needed.

Another direction for research concerns the question of side effects, which are sometimes so intense that they can lead patients to stop their treatment or slow their dosage increases. The answer to this question may lie in the development of medications that activate GABA-B receptors differently than baclofen in a way that produces fewer side effects.

Finally, in a very different direction, it could be important to work on the question of the patients' voices and the need to consider more carefully the positive patient reports of their experiences with baclofen. When 10,000 patients say that they have been cured or greatly improved by a given treatment, their voices should be heard by health authorities, because these voices may possibly produce an argument of greater value than any clinical study.

References

1. Kopp P. Social cost of substance use in France [Le coût social des drogues en France]. OFDT (Note 2015-04), 2015. In French.
2. Anderson P, Møller L, Galea G. Alcohol in the European Union: Consumption, Harm and Policy Approaches. Copenhagen: World Health Organization Regional Office for Europe, 2012. Available at: http://www.euro.who.int/__data/assets/pdf_file/0003/160680/e96457.pdf. Accessed December 18, 2016.
3. Cott J, Carlsson A, Engel J, Lindqvist M. Suppression of ethanol-induced locomotor stimulation by GABA-like drugs. *Naunyn Schmiedebergs Arch Pharmacol.* 1976;295:203-9.
4. Daoust M, Saligaut C, Lhuintre JP, Moore N, Flipo JL, Boismare F. GABA transmission, but not benzodiazepine receptor stimulation, modulates ethanol intake by rats. *Alcohol.* 1987;4:469-72.
5. Kalivas PW, Stewart J. Dopamine transmission in the initiation and express of drug-and-stress-induced sensitization of motor activity. *Brain Res Brain Res Rev.* 1991;16:223–44.
6. Roberts DCS, Andrews MM, Vickers GJ. Baclofen attenuates the reinforcing effects of cocaine in rats. *Neuropsychopharmacology.* 1996;14:1-7.
7. Colombo G, Serra S, Brunetti G, et al. The GABA(B) receptor agonists baclofen and CGP 44532 prevent acquisition of alcohol drinking behaviour in alcohol-preferring rats. *Alcohol.* 2002;37:499-503.
8. Gallimberti L, Fern M, Ferrara SD, Fadda F, Gessa GL. Gamma-hydroxybutyric acid in the treatment of alcohol dependence: a double-blind study. *Alcohol Clin*

Exp Res. 1992;16:673-676.

9. Galloway GP, Frederick SL, Staggers FE Jr, Gonzales M, Stalcup SA, Smith DE. Gamma-hydroxybutyrate: an emerging drug of abuse that causes physical dependence. *Addiction.* 1997;92:89-96.

10. Oliveto A, Gentry WB, Pruzinsky R, Gonsai K, Kosten TR, Martell B, Poling J. Behavioral effects of gamma-hydroxybutyrate in humans. *Behav Pharmacol.* 2010;21:332-42.

11. Addolorato G, Caputo F, Capristo E, Colombo G, Gessa GL, Gasbarrini G. Ability of baclofen in reducing alcohol craving and intake: II—Preliminary clinical evidence. *Alcohol Clin Exp Res.* 2000;24:67-71.

12. Addolorato G, Caputo F, Capristo E, et al. Baclofen efficacy in reducing alcohol craving and intake: a preliminary double-blind randomized controlled study. *Alcohol.* 2002;37:504-508.

13. Addolorato G, Leggio L, Ferrulli A, et al. Effectiveness and safety of baclofen for maintenance of alcohol abstinence in alcohol-dependent patients with liver cirrhosis: randomised, double-blind controlled study. *Lancet.* 2007;370:1915-1922.

14. Addolorato G, Leggio L, Ferrulli A, et al. Baclofen Study Group. Dose-response effect of baclofen in reducing daily alcohol intake in alcohol dependence: secondary analysis of a randomized, double-blind, placebo-controlled trial. *Alcohol.* 2011;46:312-7.

15. Flannery BA, Garbutt JC, Cody MW, et al. Baclofen for alcohol dependence: A preliminary open-label study. *Alcohol Clin Exp Res.* 2004;28:1517-23.

16. Garbutt JC, Kampov-Polevoy AB, Gallop R, Kalka-Juhl L, Flannery BA. Efficacy and safety of baclofen for alcohol dependence: a randomized, double-blind, placebo-controlled trial. *Alcohol Clin Exp Res.* 2010;34:1849-1857.

17. Morley KC, Baillie A, Leung S, Addolorato G, Leggio L, Haber PS. Baclofen for the treatment of alcohol dependence and possible role of comorbid anxiety. *Alcohol.* 2014 pii: agu062. [Epub ahead of print].

18. Ponizovsky AM, Rosca P, Aronovich E, Weizman A, Grinshpoon A. Baclofen as add-on to standard psychosocial treatment for alcohol dependence: a randomized, double-blind, placebo-controlled trial with a 1-year follow-up. *J Subst Abuse Treat.* 2015;52:24-30.

19. Ameisen O. Complete and prolonged suppression of symptoms and consequences of alcohol-dependence using high-dose baclofen: a self-case report of a physician. *Alcohol.* 2005;40:147-50.

20. Agabio R, Marras P, Addolorato G, Carpiniello B, Gessa GL. Baclofen suppresses alcohol intake and craving for alcohol in a schizophrenia alcohol-dependent patient: a case report. *J Clin Psychopharmacol.* 2007;27:319-22.

21. Bucknam W. Suppression of symptoms of alcohol dependence and craving using high-dose baclofen. *Alcohol.* 2007;42:158-60.

22. Pastor A, Jones DM, Currie J. High-dose baclofen for treatment-resistant alcohol dependence. *J Clin Psychopharmacol.* 2012;32:266-8.

23. Ameisen O. Le Dernier Verre. Paris: Denoël, 2008 (English Edition: *The End of My Addiction.* New-York: Sarah Crichton Books, 2009).

24. Ameisen O, de Beaurepaire R. Suppression of alcohol dependence and alcohol consumption with high-dose baclofen: an open trial [Suppression de la dépendance à l'alcool et de la consommation d'alcool par le baclofène à haute dose: un essai en ouvert]. *Ann Méd-Psychol.* 2010;168:159-62. In French.

25. Gache P. Baclofène. *Alcohol Addictol.* 2010;32:119-24.
26. Dore GM, Lo K, Juckes L, Bezyan S, Latt N. Clinical experience with baclofen in the management of alcohol-dependent patients with psychiatric comorbidity: a selected case series. *Alcohol.* 2011;46:714-20.
27. Rigal L, Alexandre-Dubroeucq C, de Beaurepaire R, Le Jeunne C, Jaury P. Abstinence and "low-risk" consumption 1 year after the initiation of high-dose baclofen: A retrospective study among "high-risk" drinkers. *Alcohol.* 2012;47:439-42.
28. de Beaurepaire R. Suppression of alcohol dependence using baclofen: a 2-year observational study of 100 patients. *Front Psychiatry.* 2012;3:103.
29. Müller CA, Geisel O, Pelz P, Higl V, et al. High-dose baclofen for the treatment of alcohol dependence (BACLAD study): a randomized, placebo-controlled trial. *Eur Psychopharmacol.* 2015;25:1167-77.
30. Jaury P, Rigal L, Porcher R, Poignant S, et al. Bacloville: Clinical efficacy study of high-dose baclofen in reducing alcohol consumption in high-risk drinkers. ISBRA, Berlin, 2016.
31. Reynaud M, Paille F, Detilleux M, Aubin HJ. A randomized, double-blind, placebo-controlled efficacy study of high-dose baclofen in alcohol-dependent patients: The Alpadir study. ISBRA, Berlin, 2016.
32. Beraha EM, Salemink E, Goudriaan AE, et al. Baclofen for the treatment of alcohol dependence: a multicentre, randomized, double-blind controlled trial. ISBRA, Berlin, 2016.
33. de Beaurepaire R. The use of very high doses of baclofen in the treatment of alcohol dependence: a case series. *Front Psychiatry.* 2014;5:143.
34. Marsot A, Imbert B, Alvarez JC, et al. High variability in the exposure of baclofen in alcohol-dependent patients. *Alcohol Clin Exp Res.* 2014;38:316-21.
35. Smith CR, LaRocca NG, Giesser BS, Scheinberg LC. High-dose oral baclofen: experience in patients with multiple sclerosis. *Neurology.* 1991;41:1829-31.
36. Ling W, Shoptaw S, Majewska D. Baclofen as a cocaine anti-craving medication: A preliminary clinical study. *Neuropsychopharmacology.* 1998;18:403-4.
37. Shoptaw S, Yang X, Rotheram-Fuller EJ, et al. Randomized placebo-controlled trial of baclofen for cocaine dependence: preliminary effects for individuals with chronic patterns of cocaine use. *J Clin Psychiatry.* 2003;64:1440-8.
38. Kahn R, Biswas K, Childress AR, et al. Multi-center trial of baclofen for abstinence initiation in severe cocaine-dependent individuals. *Drug Alcohol Depend.* 2009;103:59-64.
39. Akhondzadeh S, Ahmadi-Abhari SA, Assadi SM, Shabestari OL, Kashani AR, Farzanehgan ZM. Double-blind randomized controlled trial of baclofen vs. clonidine in the treatment of opiates withdrawal. *J Clin Pharm Ther.* 2000;25:347-53.
40. Addolorato G, Leggio L, Abenavoli L, et al. Baclofen in the treatment of alcohol withdrawal syndrome: a comparative study vs diazepam. *Am J Med.* 2006;119:276.e13-18.
41. Stallings W, Schrader S. Baclofen as prophylaxis and treatment for alcohol withdrawal: a retrospective chart review. *J Okla State Med Assoc.* 2007;100:354-60.
42. Lyon JE, Khan RA, Gessert CE, Larson PM, Renier CM. Treating alcohol withdrawal with oral baclofen: a randomized, double-blind, placebo-controlled trial. *J Hosp Med.* 2011;6:469-74.

43. Franklin TR, Harper D, Kampman K, et al. The GABA B agonist baclofen reduces cigarette consumption in a preliminary double-blind placebo-controlled smoking reduction study. *Drug Alcohol Depend.* 2009;103:30-6.
44. Muralidharan K, Rajkumar RP, Mulla U, Nayak RB, Benegal V. Baclofen in the management of inhalant withdrawal: a case series. *Prim Care Companion J Clin Psychiatry.* 2008;10:48-51.
45. Liu J, Wang L. Baclofen for alcohol withdrawal. *Cochrane Database Syst Rev.* 2013;2:CD008502.
46. Berner LA, Bocarsly ME, Hoebel BG, Avena NM. Baclofen suppresses binge eating of pure fat but not a sugar-rich or sweet-fat diet. *Behav Pharmacol.* 2009;20:631-4.
47. Buda-Levin A, Wojnicki FH, Corwin RL. Baclofen reduces fat intake under binge-type conditions. *Physiol Behav.* 2005;86:176-84.
48. Maccioni P, Fantini N, Froestl W, Carai MA, Gessa GL, Colombo G. Specific reduction of alcohol's motivational properties by the positive allosteric modulator of the GABAB receptor, GS39783, comparison with the effect of the GABAB receptor direct agonist, baclofen. *Alcohol Clin Exp Res.* 2008;32:1558-64.
49. Tanchuck MA, Yoneyama N, Ford MM, Fretwell AM, Finn DA. Assessment of GABA-B, metabotropic glutamate, and opioid receptor involvement in an animal model of binge drinking. *Alcohol.* 2011;45:33-44.
50. Broft AI, Spanos A, Corwin RL, et al. Baclofen for binge eating: an open-label trial. *Int J Eat Disord.* 2007;40:687-91.
51. Corwin RL, Boan J, Peters KF, Ulbrecht JS. Baclofen reduces binge eating in a double-blind, placebo-controlled crossover study. *Behav Pharmacol.* 2012;23:616-25.
52. de Beaurepaire R, Joussaume B, Rapp A, Jaury P. Treatment of binge-eating with high-dose baclofen: a case series. *J Clin Psychopharmacol.* 2015;35:357-9.
53. Mirijello A, Addolorato G, D'Angelo C, et al. Baclofen in the treatment of persistent hiccup: a case series. *Int J Clin Pract.* 2013;67:918-21.
54. Greenhill C. Motility: Baclofen effective for rumination and supragastric belching in a pilot study. *Nat Rev Gastroenterol Hepatol.* 2011;9:3.
55. Blondeau K, Boecxstaens V, Rommel N, et al. Baclofen improves symptoms and reduces postprandial flow events in patients with rumination and supragastric belching. *Clin Gastroenterol Hepatol.* 2012;10:379-84.
56. Pozzi M, Piccinini L, Gallo M, Motta F, Radice S, Clementi E. Treatment of motor and behavioural symptoms in three Lesch-Nyhan patients with intrathecal baclofen. *Orphanet J Rare Dis.* 2014;9:208.
57. Rolland B, Bordet R, Cottencin O. Alcohol-dependence: the current French craze for baclofen. *Addiction.* 2012;107:848-9.
58. de Beaurepaire R, Jaury P. Is TRU murdering baclofen? [La RTU: est elle en train d'assassiner le baclofène?] *Le Flyer.* 2015;60:4-12. In French.
59. Rolland B, Deheul S, Danel T, Bordet R, Cottencin O. A case of de novo seizures following a probable interaction of high-dose baclofen with alcohol. *Alcohol.* 2012;47:577-80.
60. Geoffroy PA, Auffret M, Deheul S, Bordet R, Cottencin O, Rolland B. Baclofen-induced manic symptoms: case report and systematic review. *Psychosomatics.* 2014;55:326-32.
61. Swendsen JD, Merikangas KR. The comorbidity of depression and substance use disorders. *Clin Psychol Rev.* 2000;20:173-89.

Chapter Three

Baclofen in the Treatment of Alcoholism: Effectiveness in Alcohol Craving, Drinking and Relapse Prevention

Antonio Mirijello, MD, Department of Medical Sciences, Hepatology and Gastroenterology Unit, Catholic University of Rome, Italy, and Department of Medical Sciences, IRCCS Casa Sollievo della Sofferenza, San Giovanni Rotondo, Italy; Lorenzo Leggio, MD, Section on Clinical Psychoneuroendocrinology and Neuropsychopharmacology, National Institute on Alcohol Abuse and Alcoholism and National Institute on Drug Abuse, Bethesda, MD, and the Center for Alcohol and Addiction Studies, Department of Behavioral and Social Sciences, Brown University, Providence, RI; and Giovanni Addolorato, MD, Department of Medical Sciences, Hepatology and Gastroenterology Unit, Catholic University of Rome, Italy

Alcohol abstinence, reduction in alcohol intake, and relapse prevention represent critical goals in the treatment of patients with alcohol use disorder. To achieve these outcomes, the most effective strategy is the combination of medications and counseling sessions.[1]

Among the medications tested in alcohol use disorder, there is a growing interest in those medications acting on the GABA-B receptors. In fact, previous research has shown how the GABA-B receptor plays an important role in controlling alcohol drinking, alcohol reinforcement (in rats), alcohol craving (in humans), and alcohol withdrawal symptoms.[2] Baclofen is a selective GABA-B receptor agonist currently approved and used to control spasticity. Animal and human research studies indicate that baclofen is highly effective in treating patients with alcohol use disorder, including alcohol withdrawal syndrome symptoms and early and long-term relapse.[3]

This chapter summarizes the animal and human research studies with baclofen in reducing alcohol drinking and craving. Work conducted with baclofen on alcohol withdrawal syndrome is reviewed in Chapter 4.

Results from animal studies

In preclinical settings, the "anti-alcohol" profile of baclofen has been investigated using different animal experimental procedures to understand how GABA-B medications work in alcohol-related behaviors.[2-4] Specifically, non-sedative doses of baclofen, as well as other GABA-B receptor agonist medications, have been found to suppress:

- the beginning of alcohol-drinking behavior in alcohol-preferring rats given the choice between 2 bottles containing either an alcohol solution or water;
- daily alcohol intake in alcohol-experienced rats (that is, rats in which the consumption of pharmacologically relevant doses of alcohol was already established before baclofen was given, representing a model of the "active drinking" phase of human alcoholism) tested under the 2-bottle choice regimen;
- the extra amount of alcohol consumed by alcohol-preferring rats after a period of alcohol abstinence, namely the "alcohol deprivation effect," which represents a model of loss of control over alcohol drinking, mimicking the episodes of alcohol relapse in alcoholic patients;
- the increase in alcohol intake induced in alcohol-preferring rats by the administration of opioid (narcotic) and cannabinoid (marijuana-derived) drugs;
- oral self-administration (drinking) of alcohol in rats trained to press a lever to get alcohol;
- the motivational properties of alcohol in rats, measured by the extinction response procedure (that is, the maximum amount of "work" that rats trained to press a lever for alcohol are willing to perform to obtain alcohol [a validated experimental model of craving for alcohol]);
- the development of tolerance to the effects of alcohol, on balance, in mice tested on a rotating drum;
- the severity of different signs of alcohol withdrawal syndrome in rats made physically dependent on alcohol; and
- alcohol-induced stimulation of locomotor activity (that is, the animal correlate of alcohol's euphoria-inducing properties) in mice.

With regard to how baclofen works to reduce alcohol consumption and alcohol's motivational and reinforcing properties, microdialysis (a minimally invasive sampling technique) experiments showed that baclofen suppressed alcohol-stimulated dopamine release in the brains of rats.[2] Experimental evidence suggests that nerve cells in the brain, called mesolimbic dopamine neurons, are involved in the mediation of alcohol intake and reinforcement.[4]

GABA-B receptors are located in the ventral tegmental area of the brain (the area where mesolimbic dopamine neurons originate), both on the cell body of dopamine neurons and on the terminals of glutamatergic afferent neurons. Their activation by GABA-B receptor agonist medications may inhibit the dopamine neurons, which may be how baclofen suppresses alcohol-stimulated dopamine release and, in turn, dopamine-mediated alcohol-reinforced and alcohol-motivated behaviors.

Finally, some experts think that baclofen-induced activation of GABA-B receptors might counterbalance the enhanced N-methyl-D-aspartate (NMDA)–mediated glutamate excitatory neurotransmission that occurs with alcohol withdrawal syndrome, resulting in fewer or less severe symptoms of alcohol withdrawal.

Results from clinical studies

The first open-label, 4-week pilot study with 10 alcoholic men showed that baclofen (10 mg 3 times a day after a 3-day dose adjustment) in addition to weekly counseling sessions reduced alcohol craving and intake.[5] Of the 9 patients who completed the study, 7 stayed completely abstinent from alcohol, and 2 substantially reduced the amount they drank each day during the treatment period. A significant reduction in craving was observed from the first week of treatment.

These encouraging results led the same team of researchers to look into the effectiveness of baclofen in a randomized, double-blind, placebo-controlled study.[6] Baclofen or a placebo was administered for 4 weeks to 39 alcohol-dependent patients who were not hospitalized. In addition to weekly counseling sessions, participants received 10 mg of baclofen or placebo 3 times a day after a 3-day dose adjustment.

Patients treated with baclofen achieved and stayed abstinent from alcohol in a significantly higher percentage (70%) than in the placebo group (21.1%). In addition, the drop-out rate was lower among the baclofen group (15%) than in the placebo group (42.1%). A significant reduction of daily alcohol intake, an increase of total abstinence, and a reduction of all alcohol craving scores, as measured by the Obsessive Compulsive Drinking Scale, were found in the baclofen group with respect to the placebo group. Furthermore, there was a significant reduction in anxiety, as measured by the State and Trait Inventory Scale, in the baclofen group compared with the placebo group.[6]

A subsequent open-label pilot study was conducted by researchers Flannery and colleagues.[7] In this study, 9 men and 3 women were enrolled in a 12-week study using 10 mg of baclofen 3 times a day in addition to 4 sessions of talk therapy. Although only 30% of the participants completed the entire 12-week period, the number of drinks per drinking day, the number of heavy drinking days, and craving and anxiety scores were significantly reduced. Moreover, there was an increase in the number of abstinent days.

More recently, other open-label studies with baclofen have confirmed the ability of the drug to reduce alcohol craving and intake, thus promoting alcohol abstinence, as well as the ability of baclofen to reduce anxiety.[8–10] Interestingly, these studies also showed a reduction of stress hormones related to the hypothalamic-pituitary-adrenal axis, such as cortisol[9] and aldosterone.[10] These findings suggest that the hypothalamic-pituitary axis might be involved in the actions of baclofen related to the central nervous system.

Two larger double-blind, placebo-controlled, randomized clinical trials with baclofen have been conducted in Italy and in the United States. Based on the safety profile of baclofen, and considering that baclofen is excreted from the body by the kidneys and is metabolized only marginally by the liver, the Italian study was conducted in alcoholic patients with cirrhosis (scarring) of the liver.[11] Inclusion criteria consisted of both a current diagnosis of alcohol dependence and a diagnosis of cirrhosis of the liver, a group usually excluded from alcohol medication trials because of the risk that the medications could worsen the liver disease. In this randomized, controlled trial, baclofen (10 mg 3 times a day) or placebo was administered for a 12-week period in addition to counseling and medical management at each clinic visit.

In this study, baclofen showed a significant positive effect, compared with placebo, in reducing alcohol drinking and craving. In particular, a significantly higher percentage of patients treated with baclofen achieved and maintained total alcohol abstinence. Cumulative abstinence durations (CAD) were significantly higher in the baclofen group than in the placebo group. Survival analysis revealed a significantly greater chance in the baclofen group of remaining free of lapse and relapse to alcohol consumption. The number of dropouts was higher in the placebo group than in the baclofen group. A significant reduction of all alcohol craving scores was found in the baclofen group compared with the placebo group. No serious side effects leading any patients to stop the drug were reported, and no patient discontinued treatment because of a side effect.

No patient showed hyperammonemia (excess ammonia in the blood) and/or encephalopathy (a disease that results in abnormal brain structure or function) during the study, and all patients tolerated the baclofen fairly well. This study was the first to suggest the high safety, tolerability, and effectiveness of baclofen in alcoholic patients with severe alcohol use disorder, as reflected by the presence of severe liver damage.[11] Similar results were found in a subset of alcoholic patients with cirrhosis of the liver and hepatitis C.[12]

The safety of baclofen in the treatment of alcoholic patients with clinically significant liver damage was subsequently confirmed by other researchers.[13,14] Baclofen was recently included in both the European Association for the Study of the Liver[15] and the American Association for the Study of Liver Diseases[16] guidelines on the management of alcoholic liver disease.

In the randomized, controlled trial in the United States, 80 alcohol-dependent patients were treated with either 10 mg of baclofen 3 times a day or placebo for 12 weeks.[17] Both groups of patients also received 9 sessions of a counseling intervention called BRENDA over the 12-week period. This study showed a significant overall positive treatment effect: a 43% reduction in the percentage of heavy drinking days and a 37% increase in the percentage of days abstinent from alcohol.

However, this trial failed to find any significant difference between baclofen and placebo on either percentage of heavy drinking days or days abstinent from alcohol. No difference in craving scores, tested by the Penn Alcohol Craving Scale, or anxiety was found between the baclofen and placebo groups. In this study, a very high placebo effect was found, and this factor could have affected the ability of the trial to detect a baclofen effect, as the researchers noted. A placebo effect occurs when people given a placebo rather than the study drug derive a benefit from it based on their belief in its effectiveness.

The datasets of the first study[6] and of the U.S. randomized, controlled trial were compared,[18] and some baseline differences might explain the basis of the contrasting results. In particular, subjects enrolled in the Italian randomized, controlled trial showed higher alcohol consumption, more withdrawal symptoms, and higher anxiety scores than the subjects in the United

States. In summary, the majority of the studies support the high effectiveness of baclofen in patients with alcohol use disorder. Differences in patient populations, particularly in the severity of their alcohol use disorder, may explain the differences in outcomes across trials.

Finally, the International Baclofen Intervention Study was designed to test the effectiveness and tolerability of baclofen at 2 doses (10 mg or 20 mg 3 times a day) versus placebo in alcohol-dependent patients in a double-blind, randomized fashion. The targeted sample was not reached; therefore, the study was underpowered (unable) to detect an effect on the *a priori* outcomes.[19] Nonetheless, a post-hoc analysis showed a dose-response effect of baclofen, meaning that the response to baclofen was affected by the dose.[19] In particular, both doses of baclofen were significantly more effective than placebo in reducing alcohol intake. Moreover, 20 mg of baclofen 2 times a day compared with 10 mg of baclofen 3 times a day significantly reduced the number of drinks that the participants consumed per day.[20]

The safety and efficacy of baclofen has been tested in a recently published randomized, placebo-controlled U.S. trial. A total of 180 patients affected by chronic hepatitis C infection and comorbid alcohol use disorder were assigned to receive baclofen 10 mg 3 times (88) or placebo (92). In this trial, baclofen, although well tolerated, did not significantly improve CAD nor reduce heavy drinking days compared to placebo. According to the authors, this lack of efficacy could be due to the differences in patients' characteristics with respect to European Union (EU) trials: recruitment setting (hepatology clinic instead of alcohol use disorder unit), chronic outpatients instead of acute in-patients and, most of all, the low severity of alcohol use disorder at diagnosis, which could explain the high placebo response.[21]

Controversies in the treatment of alcohol use disorder with high doses of baclofen

The usefulness of baclofen for alcohol use disorder was supported, in particular in France, by several case reports, case series, and observational studies in which doses of baclofen higher than those initially used in the first studies were used.[22-27] In particular, the first self-case report by Olivier Ameisen, MD, was also described in *The End of My Addiction*, a book that had a large mass media visibility.[28]

Probably due to the pressure of the patients' association, in March 2014, the French Government Medications Agency granted a temporary recommendation to use baclofen in the treatment of alcohol use disorder. In particular, the reimbursement of the baclofen costs for the treatment of alcohol use disorder was authorized.[29] Off-label use of high doses of baclofen (that is, up to 300 mg a day or more) to treat alcohol use disorder has spread in France during the past few years.[27-31] The major criticism is that the safety of high doses has not been established via well-controlled, dose-finding, randomized, controlled trials.[30]

A recent randomized, controlled trial evaluated the effectiveness and safety of individually adjusted high doses of baclofen (30 to 270 mg a day) in a 24-week study.[32] In particular, the study period was divided into 4 phases consisting of an adjustment phase (up to 4 weeks, depending on the individually tolerated high dose), a high-dose phase (12 weeks), a tapering phase (up to 4 weeks), and a follow-up period (4 weeks after stoppage of the study medication). The dose of baclofen consumed by patients during the high-dose phase was, on average, 180 mg a day. The drug was significantly effective with respect to placebo to increase total alcohol abstinence and CAD. The drug was well tolerated, and no serious side effects were reported. No patients experienced euphoria, stimulating effects, or craving for the drug after the baclofen was stopped.

In conclusion, this study confirmed the effectiveness of baclofen in the treatment of alcohol use disorder, also showing that giving the high doses was safe.

However, a randomized controlled trial after the previously mentioned trial failed to confirm these data.[33] A total of 151 alcohol-dependent patients were enrolled to receive high-dose baclofen (58 receiving up to 150 mg a day), low-dose baclofen (31 receiving 30 mg a day), or placebo (62). In contrast with the previous randomized, controlled trial, no significant difference in baclofen, either at low dose or high dose, with respect to placebo, was found in the main outcome (time to first relapse). The researchers concluded that the lack of effectiveness could be due to differences in the treatment setting, rates of psychological support (patients were treated in the hospital for at least 28 days, with an extensive psychological support program), and patient characteristics (less severe alcohol use disorder).

More randomized, controlled trials are needed before anyone can draft definitive conclusions on the safety of high doses of baclofen in the treatment of patients with alcohol use disorder.

At the moment, the use of high-dose baclofen remains a controversial point because the use of high doses of baclofen is most likely to induce specific serious drug reactions such as overdose, baclofen withdrawal syndrome, or new-onset seizures.[29] Moreover, using high doses of baclofen for drinking reduction may sedate some patients, due to increased interactions among baclofen, alcohol, and other sedative medications.[34,35]

Researchers Imbert and colleagues recently developed and validated a model to correlate baclofen plasma (the fluid portion of the blood) concentrations and craving in a group of 67 alcohol-dependent patients. Baclofen reduced craving in all patients, but the response to baclofen was different in such a way that the researchers proposed a classification of those who responded to the drug early versus those who responded to it late.[36] Understanding these differences could lead to a tailored therapy and dosage regimen, avoiding the use of high doses of baclofen and the related risk of side effects in patients who do not need high doses.

Baclofen effectiveness in specific subtypes of patients

The concept underlying the identifications of alcohol use disorder types has evolved from the conception of alcohol use disorder as a disease state to a personality model. This model is supported by genetic epidemiological data and extended into a measure of disease severity determined through cluster (statistical) analysis, using detailed empirical (observed) data derived from hospitalized patients with alcohol use disorder.[29,38]

Patients with alcohol use disorder can also be classified on the basis of craving characteristics. [28,37,41] In particular, reward craving is characterized by a dopaminergic/opioidergic dysregulation or a characteristic personality trait defined by the search for reward and/or the need for reward. Obsessive craving (a loss of control over intrusive thoughts about drinking alcohol) is characterized by a serotoninergic dysregulation (serotonin deficit) or a personality trait consisting of disinhibition or a combination of both factors. The main characteristic of obsessive craving is loss of control.

Relief craving (desire to decrease tension) is characterized by a GABAergic/glutamatergic dysregulation or a personality trait manifesting itself through reactivity to stress or a combination of both factors. The main characteristic of this type of craving in these patients is mainly the "need for relief."

Although there are few data, it is conceivable that different medications could be more effective in different craving mechanisms and subtypes of patients, so the evaluation of each patient's type could help doctors to select the most appropriate medication.[42] In this regard, emerging data suggest that baclofen could be most useful in specific subtypes of patients. On the basis of its action on the GABA-B receptor and of the characteristics of the patients who responded to baclofen in the previous randomized, controlled trials, it has been suggested that baclofen may work better in reducing relief and obsessive cravings.[43]

More work is needed to further understand how baclofen may work to reduce alcohol consumption in patients with alcohol use disorder. As a case in point, a small, double-blind, controlled, randomized, human laboratory study was conducted with 14 alcohol-dependent, heavy-drinking patients who were not seeking treatment but who received either 10 mg of baclofen 3 times a day or an active placebo for 7 days. On day 8, an alcohol cue-reactivity procedure followed by an alcohol self-administration session was performed. The main results showed an effect of baclofen in increasing alcohol-related sedation and stimulation.

In addition, a combined variable of alcohol consumed during the alcohol self-administration period and the 2 days before showed a positive effect of baclofen in reducing alcohol drinking. Exploratory analyses tentatively suggested that anxiety, the D4 dopamine receptor DRD4 $\geq$7 repeats (DRD4L), and the -HTTLPR LL genotype moderated baclofen's effects.[44]

Researchers Morley and colleagues performed a double-blind, placebo-controlled, randomized, controlled trial with 42 alcohol-dependent patients who received 10 mg of baclofen 3 times a day or 20 mg of baclofen 3 times a day or placebo. The structured psychosocial therapy BRENDA was offered to all patients. Analyses revealed that alcohol consumption was significantly reduced among patients in all 3 groups.

However, an analysis conducted after stratifying patients by the presence or lack of a diagnosis of a co-occurring anxiety disorder indicated a beneficial effect of 10 mg of baclofen 3 times a day on time to lapse and relapse limited to those alcoholic patients with an anxiety disorder. For classification purposes, relapse is defined as a daily alcohol intake of more than 4 drinks or an overall consumption of 14 drinks or more per week during at least 4 weeks; lapse represents any episode of alcohol consumption not classified as relapse.

Moreover, in this subgroup of patients, there was a beneficial effect with 20 mg of baclofen 3 times a day compared with placebo on time to relapse to drinking. Both doses of baclofen were well tolerated, and there were no serious adverse events.[45]

Finally, given the strong relationship between alcoholism and smoking, a 12-week, double-blind, randomized, controlled trial was conducted to examine the role of baclofen in reducing alcohol and cigarette co-use in 30 alcoholic smokers seeking treatment for both conditions. Baclofen, compared with placebo, increased the percentage of days of abstinence from both alcohol and tobacco, although it did not reduce the percentage of days of co-use. The severity of alcohol dependence moderated, or changed, the baclofen response. In fact, those patients with the most severe alcohol dependence and who were treated with baclofen had the largest increase in the percentage of days of abstinence from both alcohol and tobacco.[46]

Conclusions

Baclofen represents a promising drug for the treatment of alcohol use disorder. In view of its safety and tolerability and considering the data summarized above, baclofen may be the drug of choice for the treatment of specific types of patients, including patients with such severe comorbidities as advanced liver damage, who are usually excluded from drug treatments for alcohol use disorder because most are metabolized through the liver.

Finally, given the effectiveness of this drug in the treatment of alcohol withdrawal syndrome[47,48] (see Chapter 4), baclofen could be a useful and unique drug in the treatment of different phases of alcohol use disorder, from the detoxification stage to the long-term relapse-prevention program.

Acknowledgments

We are grateful to Drs. Anna Ferrulli, Cristina d'Angelo, Gabriele Vassallo, Mariangela Antonelli, Claudia Tarli, Filippo Bernardini and Luisa Sestito for their contribution to some of the baclofen studies conducted in our laboratory.

References

1. Addolorato G, Mirijello A, Leggio L. Alcohol addiction: toward a patient-oriented pharmacological treatment. *Expert Opin Pharmacother.* 2013; 14: 2157-60.
2. Colombo G, Addolorato G, Agabio R, et al. Role of GABA(B) receptor in alcohol dependence: reducing effect of baclofen on alcohol intake and alcohol motivational properties in rats and amelioration of alcohol withdrawal syndrome and alcohol craving in human alcoholics. *Neurotox Res.* 2004;6:403-14.
3. Johnson BA, Swift RM, Addolorato G, Ciraulo DA, Myrick H. Safety and efficacy of GABAergic medications for treating alcoholism. *Alcohol Clin Exp Res.* 2005;29:248-54.
4. Addolorato G, Leggio L, Agabio R, Colombo G, Gasbarrini G. Baclofen: a new drug for the treatment of alcohol dependence. *Int J Clin Pract.* 2006;60:1003-8.
5. Addolorato G, Caputo F, Capristo E, Colombo G, Gessa GL, Gasbarrini G. Ability of baclofen in reducing alcohol craving and intake: II—Preliminary clinical evidence. *Alcohol Clin Exp Res.* 2000;24:67-71.
6. Addolorato G, Caputo F, Capristo E, et al. Baclofen efficacy in reducing alcohol craving and intake: a preliminary double-blind randomized controlled study. *Alcohol.* 2002;37:504-8.
7. Flannery BA, Garbutt JC, Cody MW, et al. Baclofen for alcohol dependence: a preliminary open-label study. *Alcohol Clin Exp Res.* 2004;28:1517-23.
8. Leggio L, Ferrulli A, Cardone S, et al. Relationship between the hypothalamic-pituitary-thyroid axis and alcohol craving in alcohol dependent patients: a longitudinal study. *Alcohol Clin Exp Res.* 2008;32:2047-53.
9. Leggio L, Ferrulli A, Cardone S, et al. Renin and aldosterone but not the natriuretic peptide correlate with obsessive craving in medium-term abstinent alcohol-dependent patients: a longitudinal study. *Alcohol.* 2008;42:375-81.
10. Leggio L, Ferrulli A, Malandrino N, et al. Insulin but not insulin growth factor-1 correlates with craving in currently drinking alcohol-dependent patients. *Alcohol Clin Exp Res.* 2008;32:450-8.
11. Addolorato G, Leggio L, Ferrulli A, et al. Effectiveness and safety of baclofen for maintenance of alcohol abstinence in alcohol-dependent patients with liver cirrhosis: randomised, double-blind controlled study. *Lancet.* 2007;370:1915-22.
12. Leggio L, Ferrulli A, Zambon A, et al. Baclofen promotes alcohol abstinence in alcohol dependent cirrhotic patients with hepatitis C virus (HCV) infection. *Addict Behav.* 2012; 37: 561-4.
13. Heydtmann M. Baclofen effect related to liver damage. *Alcohol Clin Exp Res.* 2011;35:848.
14. Yamini D, Lee SH, Avanesyan A, Walter M, Runyon B. Utilization of baclofen in maintenance of alcohol abstinence in patients with alcohol dependence and alcoholic hepatitis with or without cirrhosis. *Alcohol* 2014; 49: 453-6.
15. European Association for the Study of the Liver. EASL clinical practical guidelines: management of alcoholic liver disease. *J Hepatol.* 2012;57:399-420.
16. Runyon BA; AASLD. Introduction to the revised American Association for the Study of Liver Diseases Practice Guideline management of adult patients with ascites due to cirrhosis 2012. *Hepatol.* 2013;57:1651-3.

17. Garbutt JC, Kampov-Polevoy AB, Gallop R, Kalka-Juhl L, Flannery BA. Efficacy and safety of baclofen for alcohol dependence: a randomized, double-blind, placebo-controlled trial. *Alcohol Clin Exp Res.* 2010;34:1849-57.
18. Leggio L, Garbutt JC, Addolorato G. Effectiveness and safety of baclofen in the treatment of alcohol-dependent patients. *CNS Neurol Disord Drug Targets.* 2010;9:33-44.
19. Addolorato G, Leggio L. Safety and efficacy of baclofen in the treatment of alcohol-dependent patients. *Curr Pharm Des.* 2010;16(19):2113-7.
20. Addolorato G, Leggio L, Ferrulli A, et al; Baclofen Study Group. Dose-response effect of baclofen in reducing daily alcohol intake in alcohol dependence: secondary analysis of a randomized, double-blind, placebo-controlled trial. *Alcohol.* 2011;46:312-7.
21. Hauser P, Fuller B, Ho SB, Thuras P, Kern S, Dieperink E. The Safety and Efficacy of Baclofen to Reduce Alcohol Use in Veterans with Chronic Hepatitis C: A Randomized Clinical Trial. *Addiction.* 2017 Feb 13. doi: 10.1111/add.13787.
22. Ameisen O. Complete and prolonged suppression of symptoms and consequences of alcohol-dependence using high-dose baclofen: a self-case report of a physician. *Alcohol.* 2005; 40: 147-50.
23. Bucknam W. Suppression of symptoms of alcohol dependence and craving using high-dose baclofen. *Alcohol.* 2007;42:158-60.
24. de Beaurepaire R. The use of very high-doses of baclofen for the treatment of alcohol dependence: a case series. *Front Psychiatry.* 2014;5:143.
25. Pastor A, Jones DM, Currie J. High-dose baclofen for treatment resistant alcohol dependence. *J Clin Psychopharmacol.* 2012;32:266-8.
26. Rigal L, Alexandre-Dubroeucq C, de Beaurepaire R, Le Jeunne C, Jaury P. Abstinence and "low-risk" consumption 1 year after the initiation of high-dose baclofen: a retrospective study among "high-risk" drinkers. *Alcohol.* 2012;47:439-42.
27. Rolland B, Paille F, Fleury B, Cottencin O, Benyamina A, Aubin HJ. Off-label baclofen prescribing practices among French alcohol specialists: results of a national online survey. *PLoS One.* 2014;9:e98062.
28. Ameisen O. *Le Dernier Verre.* Ed. Denoel 2008.
29. No author listed. Baclofen: Hope for alcoholism treatment, but more trials needed. *Alcoholism Drug Abuse Weekly.* 2014;26:Apr 7.
30. Mirijello A, Caputo F, Vassallo G, et al. GABA(B) agonists for the treatment of alcohol use disorder. *Curr Pharm Des.* 2015; 21: 3367-72.
31. Dupouy J, Fournier JP, Jouanjus É, et al. Baclofen for alcohol dependence in France: incidence of treated patients and prescription patterns: a cohort study. *Eur Neuropsychopharmacol.* 2014;24:192-9.
32. Müller CA, Geisel O, Pelz P, et al. High-dose baclofen for the treatment of alcohol dependence (BACLAD study): a randomized, placebo-controlled trial. *Eur Neuropsychopharmacol.* 2015;25:1167-77.
33. Beraha EM, Salemink E, Goudriaan AE, et al. Efficacy and safety of high-dose baclofen for the treatment of alcohol dependence: a multicentre, randomised, double-blind controlled trial. *Eur Neuropsychopharmacol.* 2016; Nov 11. pii: S0924-977X(16)31968-X. doi: 10.1016/j.euroneuro.2016.10.006.

34. Rolland B, Bordet R, Cottencin O. Alcohol-dependence: the current French craze for baclofen: *Addiction.* 2012;107:848-9.
35. Rolland B, Valin T, Langlois C, et al. Safety and drinking outcomes among patients with comorbid alcohol dependence and borderline personality disorder treated with high-dose baclofen: a comparative cohort study. *Int Clin Psychopharmacol.* 2015;30:49-53.
36. Imbert B, Alvarez JC, Simon N. Anticraving effect of baclofen in alcohol-dependent patients. *Alcohol Clin Exp Res.* 2015;39:1602-8.
37. Leggio L. Understanding and treating alcohol craving and dependence: recent pharmacological and neuroendocrinological findings. *Alcohol.* 2009;44:341-52.
38. Johnson BA. Medication treatment of different types of alcoholism. *Am J Psychiatry.* 2010;167:630-9.
39. Leggio L, Kenna GA, Fenton M, Bonenfant E, Swift RM. Typologies of alcohol dependence. From Jellinek to genetics and beyond. *Neuropsychol Rev.* 2009;19:115-29.
40. Enoch MA. Pharmacogenomics of alcohol response and addiction. *Am J Pharmacogenomics.* 2003;3:217-32.
41. Lesch OM, Dietezel M, Musalek M, Walter H, Zeiler K. The course of alcoholism. Long-term prognosis in different subtypes. *Forensic Sci International.* 1988;36:121-38.
42. Addolorato G, Leggio L, Abenavoli L, Gasbarrini G; Alcoholism Treatment Study Group. Neurobiochemical and clinical aspects of craving in alcohol addiction: a review. *Addict Behav.* 2005;30:1209-24.
43. Addolorato G, Abenavoli L, Leggio L, Gasbarrini G. How many cravings? Pharmacological aspects of craving treatment in alcohol addiction: a review. *Neuropsychobiol.* 2005;51:59-66.
44. Leggio L, Zywiak WH, McGeary JE, et al. A human laboratory pilot study with baclofen in alcoholic individuals. *Pharmacol Biochem Behav.* 2013;103:784-91.
45. Morley KC, Baillie A, Leung S, Addolorato G, Leggio L, Haber PS. Baclofen for the treatment of alcohol dependence and possible role of comorbid anxiety. *Alcohol.* 2014. pii: agu062.
46. Leggio L, Zywiak WH, Edwards SM, Tidey JW, Swift RM, Kenna GA. A preliminary double-blind, placebo-controlled randomized study of baclofen effects in alcoholic smokers. *Psychopharmacology* (Berl). 2015;232:233-43.
47. Addolorato G, Leggio L, Abenavoli L, et al. Baclofen in the treatment of alcohol withdrawal syndrome: a comparative study vs diazepam. *Am J Med.* 2006;119:276.e13-8.
48. Mirijello A, D'Angelo C, Ferrulli A, et al. Identification and management of alcohol withdrawal syndrome. *Drugs.* 2015;75:353-65.

Chapter Four

The Role of Baclofen in the Treatment of Alcohol Withdrawal Syndrome

Mehdi Farokhnia, MD, Section on Clinical Psychoneuroendocrinology and Neuropsychopharmacology, National Institute on Alcohol Abuse and Alcoholism and National Institute on Drug Abuse, National Institutes of Health, Bethesda, Maryland; Giovanni Addolorato, MD, Department of Internal Medicine, Catholic University of Rome, Gemelli Hospital, Rome, Italy; and Lorenzo Leggio, MD, PhD, MSc, Section on Clinical Psychoneuroendocrinology and Neuropsychopharmacology, National Institute on Alcohol Abuse and Alcoholism and National Institute on Drug Abuse, National Institutes of Health, Bethesda, Maryland and the Center for Alcohol and Addiction Studies, Department of Behavioral and Social Sciences, Brown University, Providence, Rhode Island

In this chapter, we review the research on the use of baclofen for the treatment of alcohol withdrawal syndrome. Baclofen's effects on alcohol drinking and craving are reviewed in Chapter 3.

Withdrawal from alcohol: definition, neurobiology and management

What is alcohol withdrawal syndrome?

Alcohol withdrawal syndrome is a set of signs and symptoms that may develop after significantly decreasing the amount of alcohol usually consumed or abruptly stopping drinking. Many alcohol-dependent patients experience some degree of withdrawal symptoms at some point during the course of their disease. This is a major source of distress to patients and significantly limits their ability to stop drinking.[1,2]

Prompt diagnosis and treatment is critical because alcohol withdrawal syndrome is a preventable cause of illness and death and can be a life-threatening condition in its most severe forms.[3] Notably, physiological adaptation to alcohol may make even some non-dependent patients susceptible to withdrawal symptoms when they are hospitalized for any reason (because they no longer have access to alcohol), an event that increases the complexity and cost of their hospitalization.[4,5]

Alcohol withdrawal syndrome presents in different forms with a wide range of signs and symptoms. Mild-to-moderate symptoms usually start 6 to 24 hours after the last drink and include hand tremor (involuntary shaking), sweating, restlessness, agitation, anxiety, depression, fever, high blood pressure, fast heart rate, rapid breathing, nausea, vomiting, and sleep problems. In more severe forms, some patients may hear, see, or feel things that aren't there (hallucinations).

Complicated alcohol withdrawal syndrome typically develops 24 to 72 hours after the last alcoholic drink and includes generalized tonic–clonic seizure, delirium tremens, or both.[3] Generalized tonic-clonic seizure is a convulsion in which a person loses consciousness, their muscles stiffen, and they make jerking movements. Delirium tremens is a medical emergency characterized by prominent disturbances in attention, cognition, perception, and orientation. These signs change rapidly and can occur with mood swings, psychomotor agitation (for example, wringing of the hands, pacing around the room), periods of intense sweating, fever, high blood pressure, rapid and/or irregular heartbeat, and respiratory complications (for example, rapid and shallow breathing).[6,7] Cardiac arrest and death has been reported in 5% to 10% of patients with complicated alcohol withdrawal syndrome.[8,9]

Alcohol withdrawal syndrome can be diagnosed according to the standard criteria defined by the *Diagnostic and Statistical Manual of Mental Disorders (DSM);*[10] for more details, see Box 1.

Box 1. *Diagnostic and Statistical Manual of Mental Disorders (DSM)* **and Alcohol Withdrawal Syndrome**[10]

DSM is the standard classification of mental disorders, a common language used by physicians, researchers, and other mental health professionals. For each disorder, a set of criteria is indicated to make a specific diagnosis. According to *DSM-5* (the latest version of *DSM*), the diagnostic criteria of alcohol withdrawal include:

A. Cessation of (or reduction in) alcohol use that has been heavy and prolonged.

B. Two (or more) of the following, developing within several hours to a few days after the cessation of (or reduction in) alcohol use described in Criterion A:

  1. Autonomic hyperactivity (for example, sweating or pulse rate greater than 100 beats per minute)

  2. Increased hand tremor

  3. Insomnia

  4. Nausea or vomiting

  5. Transient visual, tactile, or auditory hallucinations or illusions

  6. Psychomotor agitation

  7. Anxiety

  8. Generalized tonic-clonic seizures

C. The signs or symptoms in Criterion B cause clinically significant distress or impairment in social, occupational, or other important areas of functioning.

D. The signs or symptoms are not attributable to another medical condition and are not better explained by another mental disorder, including intoxication or withdrawal from another substance.

Reprinted with permission from the *Diagnostic and Statistical Manual of Mental Disorders,* Fifth Edition, (Copyright ©2013). American Psychiatric Association. All Rights Reserved.

How does alcohol withdrawal syndrome occur?

Recent advances in neuroscience have shed light on the neurobiology of alcohol withdrawal syndrome, which means what parts of the nervous system are involved in this condition. Under normal conditions, there is a balance between inhibitory and excitatory neurotransmission, an essential balance for the brain's normal functioning. Gamma-aminobutyric acid (GABA) is the main inhibitory neurotransmitter, and glutamate is the main excitatory neurotransmitter, in the central nervous system. Throughout the brain, there are different classes of GABA and glutamate receptors (molecules that receive chemical messages and facilitate communication between the cell and outside) that play important roles in both physiological (normal) and pathological (disease) processes.[11]

In the short term, drinking alcohol causes central nervous system depression through activation of the GABAergic system and deactivation of the glutamatergic system. Alcohol's depressant effects occur as the result of stimulation of the GABA-A receptors and inhibition of the glutamate N-methyl-D-aspartate (NMDA) receptors.

Long-term alcohol consumption results in adaptive changes in an attempt to restore the equilibrium between these neurotransmitter systems. As a result, the number and function of receptors is decreased for GABA (down-regulation) and increased for glutamate (upregulation) after chronic exposure to alcohol.[12,13] These adaptive changes are responsible for the central nervous system hyperexcitability that occurs after abrupt stoppage of alcohol consumption (see Figure 1).

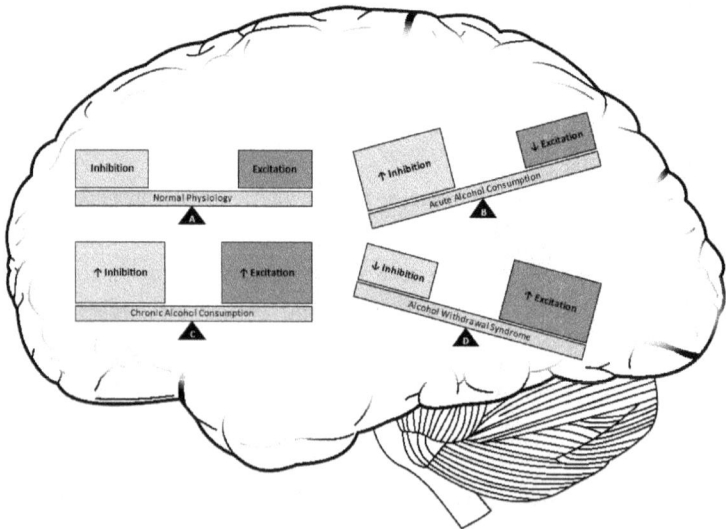

FIGURE 1. The balance of inhibitory and excitatory neurotransmission in normal physiological conditions (A), acute (short-term) alcohol consumption (B), chronic (long-term) alcohol consumption (C), and alcohol withdrawal syndrome (D).

As discussed previously, alcohol withdrawal syndrome is associated with various signs and symptoms that occur as the result of changes in different brain pathways. In addition to GABA and glutamate, several other neurotransmitters are involved in the pathophysiology (disease process) of alcohol withdrawal syndrome. For example, upregulation of the dopaminergic and noradrenergic pathways are thought to be responsible for withdrawal-induced hallucinations and autonomic hyperactivity, respectively.[2,14]

How is alcohol withdrawal syndrome treated?

Proper treatment of alcohol withdrawal syndrome is of the utmost importance. The first and main goal is to prevent the progression from mild-to-moderate symptoms to more severe and complicated forms of alcohol withdrawal syndrome. Experiencing fewer withdrawal symptoms also motivates alcohol-dependent patients to stop drinking alcohol and to stay sober as a long-term goal.

Minor withdrawal symptoms can be self-managed or treated in outpatient settings (for example, a clinic), while more severe forms require hospitalization and close monitoring.[15,16] Interventions with and without a drug are the mainstays of alcohol withdrawal syndrome treatment. Frequent reassurance, reality orientation, and a dark and quiet environment can be helpful as a first step.[17]

Currently, benzodiazepine drugs are the gold-standard medications for treating alcohol withdrawal syndrome, with chlordiazepoxide, diazepam, and lorazepam being the most commonly prescribed for this purpose.[18,19] By activating the GABA-A receptors, these medications mimic alcohol's effects, which seems to be the main way they work in reducing alcohol withdrawal symptoms.[20] However, benzodiazepines are not considered an ideal drug category for treating alcohol withdrawal syndrome, mainly because of their side effects and also because they can be addictive.[18,21,22]

The importance of treating alcohol withdrawal syndrome, along with the disadvantages of benzodiazepines, have encouraged many researchers and doctors to look into new drug options for alcohol withdrawal syndrome. The ideal medication for alcohol withdrawal syndrome should have some important qualities:

1) It should be safe, with no or few serious side effects;
2) Its metabolism should be independent of liver function because most alcohol-dependent patients have some degree of liver disease;

3) It should neither interact with alcohol nor have a potential for abuse or dependence;

4) It should have both a rapid onset and a long duration of action; and

5) In addition to relieving alcohol withdrawal symptoms, the ideal drug would also reduce alcohol craving and drinking.[3]

Consistent with these criteria, non-benzodiazepine GABAergic drugs have recently been studied as promising treatments for alcohol withdrawal syndrome, including baclofen, topiramate, gabapentin, carbamazepine, valproic acid, gamma-hydroxybutyrate, oxcarbazepine, flumazenil, tiagabine, vigabatrin, and others.[23]

Compared with benzodiazepines, most of these drugs have fewer and milder side effects, are less addictive, involve low or no liver metabolism, and are excreted mainly through the kidneys. In addition to easing withdrawal symptoms, some of these drugs may also help prevent people from returning to drinking and reduce alcohol drinking and craving.[24]

Among non-benzodiazepine GABAergic medications, the selective GABA-B receptor agonist baclofen has been looked at as a potentially effective medication for the treatment of alcohol withdrawal syndrome. Baclofen was introduced in the 1960s and approved by the U.S. Food and Drug Administration in 1977 for treating muscle spasticity (continuous contraction) associated with some neurological disorders.[25] It is thought that baclofen's inhibitory effects through activation of the GABA-B receptors might counterbalance the underlying increase in excitatory neurotransmission present during alcohol withdrawal syndrome, resulting in a reduction of withdrawal symptoms.[23,26]

Baclofen as a treatment for alcohol withdrawal syndrome

Animal studies

Before testing a new medication in humans, researchers conduct experiments in small numbers of animals to gather information on the safety and early effectiveness of a drug. The first study on the potential use of baclofen for alcohol withdrawal syndrome was published in 1980, when the researchers Tarika and Winger made 4 rhesus monkeys physically dependent on alcohol by giving them ethanol intravenously, then withdrew them from ethanol and observed alcohol withdrawal signs, including muscle weakness, ataxia (a lack of control over the muscles during voluntary movements such as walking), and tremor. A muscle injection of baclofen given 12 hours after the last alcohol injection was able to slightly reduce withdrawal-induced tremors in this experiment. However, this effect was accompanied by considerable sedation and muscle weakness and was not strong enough to allow researchers to draw definitive conclusions.[27]

A decade later, another group of researchers conducted 2 studies in ethanol-treated rats and control (not ethanol-treated) rats and showed that intraperitoneal injection of small doses of baclofen significantly reversed tremors, aggression, and anxiety-like behaviors in alcohol-withdrawn rats without having considerable sedative effects, and these effects were dose-dependent (the higher the dose, the better it relieved the signs, and vice versa).[28,29]

In contrast, a few years later, the researchers Humeniuk and colleagues showed that baclofen did not improve withdrawal signs (tremor and tail arch) and even induced convulsions (sudden involuntary movements of a limb or other part of the body) in mice that had been withdrawn from alcohol.[30]

In a comprehensive set of experiments published in 2000, researchers Colombo and colleagues assessed the effectiveness of baclofen in reducing alcohol withdrawal signs in rats made physically dependent on alcohol. Fifteen hours after the last ethanol administration, 32 rats were placed in 4 groups to receive an intraperitoneal injection of baclofen (0, 10, 20, or 40 mg/kg). The intensity of withdrawal signs was rated every hour using an 11-item scale.[31]

In this experiment, baclofen significantly relieved the alcohol withdrawal signs in a dose-dependent fashion (see Figure 2), meaning that the higher the dose, the better it relieved the signs, and vice versa. While the highest dose (40 mg/kg) caused pronounced sedation, 20 mg/kg of baclofen was well tolerated with no significant muscle weakness or loss of alertness.

In a separate experiment, 20 mg/kg of baclofen was also effective in preventing sound-induced seizures after exposing the alcohol-withdrawn rats to 30 seconds of repeated auditory stimuli (noises).[26] These results were similar to the results of previous research on the protective effects of baclofen against alcohol withdrawal seizures in rats.[32]

Later in 2007, researchers Knapp and colleagues reported that baclofen was able to prevent the expression and sensitization of anxiety-like behavior during a number of repeated ethanol-sensitization protocols. Rats were exposed to different cycles and combinations of an ethanol diet, withdrawal and stress, and the effect of several drugs on their behavior was assessed using a social interaction test. In these experiments, baclofen reduced both the

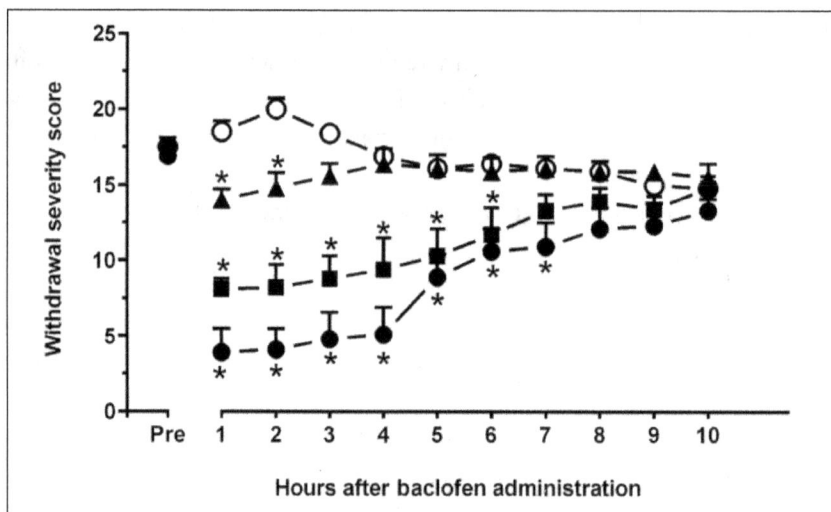

FIGURE 2. Effect of baclofen on intensity of alcohol withdrawal syndrome signs in ethanol-dependent Wistar rats.

Each point is the mean ± standard error.

Baclofen dosage key:
open circles   0 mg/kg
triangles   10 mg/kg
squares   20 mg/kg
closed circles   40 mg/kg
* statistically significant results in comparison to rats treated with saline

Reprinted from *Alcoholism: Clinical and Experimental Research*, 24/1, Giancarlo Colombo, Roberta Agabio, Mauro AM Carai, Carla Lobina, Marialaura Pani, Roberta Reali, Giovanni Addolorato, Gian Luigi Gessa, Ability of Baclofen in Reducing Alcohol Intake and Withdrawal Severity: I—Preclinical Evidence, 58-66, Copyright © 2006, with permission from John Wiley and Sons.

expression and the sensitization of the anxiety-like behavior after repeated withdrawals from alcohol.[33]

The design of this study is particularly relevant to its use in humans because it models the sensitization of withdrawal symptoms in alcoholic patients, which is called "kindling." Kindling represents long-term changes in the brain (for example, increased excitability of neurons) as a result of repeated episodes of alcohol withdrawal syndrome. It has been shown that the severity and consequences of alcohol withdrawal syndrome worsen after each episode, leading to a vicious cycle of alcohol abuse and an increased risk of more severe forms of alcohol withdrawal syndrome.[34,35]

Human studies

The promising animal work mentioned previously led researchers to further investigate if baclofen could be a safe and effective medication for treating alcohol withdrawal syndrome in alcoholic patients. A summary of such clinical studies is outlined next.

Initial reports

In a small, open-label, uncontrolled study (a study where there is no placebo and both the research subject and the researcher know which drug is being given) published in 2002, baclofen's effect was tested in 5 alcohol-dependent patients with severe alcohol withdrawal syndrome. The intensity of withdrawal symptoms was measured by a scale called the Clinical Institute Withdrawal Assessment for Alcohol (CIWA-A) (revised version) (for more details, see reference 36 and Box 1).

All 5 patients in this study had a high withdrawal score requiring drug treatment and were given a 10 mg baclofen pill after they were hospitalized. This single baclofen dose resulted in rapid reduction of withdrawal symptoms, and all patients were sent home from the hospital within 8 hours after baclofen administration.

For the next 30 days, patients were given 30 mg a day of baclofen (10 mg every 8 hours), and their withdrawal symptoms were regularly assessed as outpatients. While all patients did not drink alcohol during this period, they did not report any discomfort or withdrawal symptoms. In terms of safety, 3 patients reported mild sedation after taking baclofen. Overall, baclofen was well tolerated, and no serious side effect was reported.[37]

Later, a case report was published describing successful treatment of a patient hospitalized in an inpatient unit for delirium tremens with baclofen (25 mg 3 times a day). However, the single patient in this case was treated in a well-controlled research setting with close observation, and the results may not be applied to other settings without further investigation.[38]

More evidence of the potential role of baclofen in treating alcohol withdrawal syndrome came from a retrospective (backward-looking) review of the medical records of 42 hospitalized patients determined to be at risk for alcohol withdrawal syndrome. The results showed that baclofen prevented alcohol withdrawal syndrome in 86% of patients.[39] These results highlight not only the therapeutic uses but also the preventive potential of baclofen in the management of alcohol withdrawal syndrome. While the retrospective nature of this study represents an important limitation, this is a potentially valuable study.

In fact, many patients hospitalized in general medical or surgical wards are at increased risk for alcohol withdrawal symptoms and complications because they have stopped drinking suddenly and cannot access alcohol in the hospital. Early identification of these patients and subsequent prevention is very important because it can prevent the development of alcohol withdrawal syndrome and its potentially harmful consequences.[4,40]

> **Box 2. Clinical Institute Withdrawal Assessment for Alcohol**
> The CIWA-A[41,42] is a reliable and validated 15-item scale that has emerged as a useful tool to assess the severity of alcohol withdrawal syndrome, especially in the shortened revised form (CIWA-Ar). CIWA-Ar measures 10 signs and symptoms:
> - Nausea and vomiting
> - Tremor
> - Paroxysmal sweats
> - Anxiety
> - Agitation
> - Tactile (touch) disturbances
> - Auditory (hearing) disturbances
> - Visual (seeing) disturbances
> - Headache or a feeling of fullness in the head
> - Problems with orientation and clouding of the senses
>
> With the instructions provided, each item is scored on a scale of 0 to 7, except for the last item, which can receive a score of 0 to 4. Therefore, the highest possible CIWA-Ar score is 67.
>
> Estimating the severity of alcohol withdrawal syndrome with the CIWA-Ar can also be helpful in defining the drug treatment plan:

Table 1. Severity of alcohol withdrawal syndrome[41]			
Description	CIWA-Ar score*	Treatment setting	Pharmacological treatment
Mild	Less than 8	Outpatient (clinic)	Not indicated
Moderate	8 to 15	Outpatient (clinic) or inpatient (hospital)	Indicated (with oral medications)
Severe	More than 15	Inpatient (hospital)	Strongly indicated (with intravenous medications)
*The CIWA-Ar is not copyrighted and may be used freely.			

Preliminary controlled studies

Randomized, double-blind, placebo-controlled studies (studies where subjects are randomly given medication or a placebo but neither the researcher nor the research subject knows which one they are getting) are generally considered the gold standard of study design, providing the strongest evidence and comprehensive information about the effectiveness of a drug. However, given that benzodiazepines are effective medications for treating alcohol withdrawal syndrome, it may not be ethically justified to use placebo alone in studying new drugs for this purpose. Therefore, researchers should either use a comparative non-inferiority design (a study to show that a new treatment is not less effective than the usual treatment)[43] or test the new medication versus placebo as an add-on to the standard treatment.[42]

The initial promising clinical results led to the first randomized study in 2006, in which researchers Addolorato and colleagues compared the usefulness of baclofen with a benzodiazepine drug in the treatment of alcohol withdrawal syndrome. Thirty-seven alcohol-dependent individuals with uncomplicated moderate-to-severe alcohol withdrawal syndrome were randomly assigned to receive 1 of the 2 oral regimens for 10 days: baclofen (30 mg a day) or diazepam (0.5 to 0.75 mg/kg a day, with a 25% daily reduction from day 7 to day 10).

During this study, the severity of the alcohol withdrawal symptoms was assessed by the CIWA-Ar, and the researchers who rated this scale did not know who was being given baclofen or diazepam. The results showed that both baclofen and diazepam improved withdrawal symptoms, as indicated by comparable reduction of CIWA-Ar scores among the 2 groups (see Figure 3). However, baclofen was slightly slower than diazepam in reducing the agitation scores. In terms of safety, neither baclofen-treated nor diazepam-treated patients experienced significant side effects during the course of this study.[43]

It is important to keep in mind that only patients with no complications were enrolled in this study. Benzodiazepines remain the gold standard of treatment because they are the only class of medication with proven effectiveness in preventing alcohol withdrawal syndrome complications (seizures and delirium tremens).[18]

The first randomized, double-blind, placebo-controlled trial and the only one so far looking at baclofen's role in the treatment of alcohol withdrawal syndrome was conducted in 2011 in 2 hospitals in Duluth, Minnesota. Patients hospitalized for any reason and judged to be at risk for alcohol withdrawal syndrome were considered for participation in this study. Hospitalized patients who developed alcohol withdrawal syndrome (based on *DSM-IV* criteria) severe enough to require medication (CIWA-Ar score of 10 or higher) were put on a standard protocol of benzodiazepine treatment with lorazepam. In addition to the benzodiazepine therapy, patients were randomly assigned to receive add-on therapy with either baclofen (30 mg a day) or placebo for 3 days. Of 79 individuals who were monitored, 44 patients developed alcohol withdrawal syndrome, requiring drug treatment, and 31 (18 received baclofen, 13 received placebo) completed the full assessments of this study.

The results showed that, while the severity of alcohol withdrawal syndrome (based on CIWA-Ar scores) was similarly decreased across the groups, there was a significant difference between the 2 treatments (baclofen versus placebo) in terms of the need for high doses of lorazepam (defined as 20 mg or more during the first 72 hours). Eight patients received high-dose lorazepam, among which only 1 patient was treated with baclofen, while 7 patients received placebo.

In summary, this study suggested that adding baclofen to the treatment regimen might be an effective way to reduce the use of a high-dose benzodiazepine in the management of alcohol withdrawal syndrome.[44]

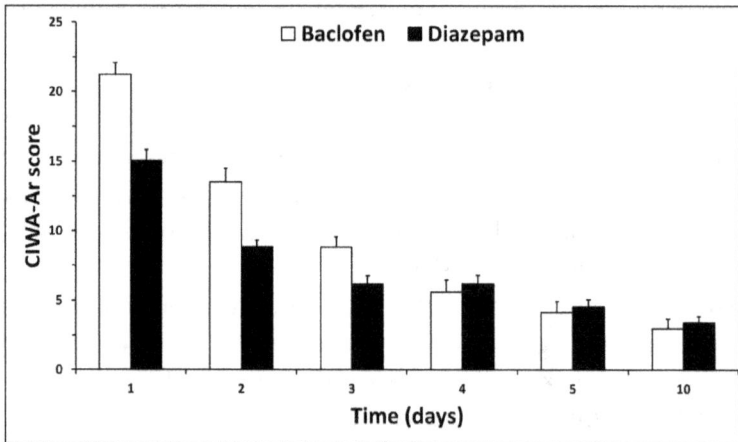

FIGURE 3. Score of the Clinical Institute Withdrawal Assessment for Alcohol–revised (CIWA-Ar) scale in patients treated for 10 consecutive days with baclofen or diazepam.

Reprinted from *The American Journal of Medicine,* 119/3, Giovanni Addolorato, Lorenzo Leggio, Ludovico Abenavoli, Roberta Agabio, Fabio Caputo, Esmeralda Capristo, Giancarlo Colombo, Gian Luigi Gessa, Giovanni Gasbarrini, Baclofen in the Treatment of Alcohol Withdrawal Syndrome: A Comparative Study vs Diazepam, 276.e13–276.e18, Copyright © 2006, with permission from Elsevier.

In general, there are 2 strategies for using medications to treat alcohol withdrawal syndrome: symptom-triggered dosing and fixed dosing. Symptom-triggered dosing is a dynamic process during which repeated measurements of CIWA-Ar (severity of alcohol withdrawal) are used to define the "as-needed" medication dosage. This approach is preferred over fixed dosing because it reduces the intensity and length of treatment as well as the total dose of benzodiazepine needed to control the alcohol withdrawal symptoms.[19,43]

Considering the potentially harmful consequences of benzodiazepine treatment, especially in high doses, many researchers have tried to explore other ways, such as add-on medications, to reduce the need for high-dose benzodiazepines. This last study mentioned is an example of a successful endeavor in this regard, in which researchers showed that baclofen was better than placebo in reducing the need for high doses of benzodiazepines in treating patients with alcohol withdrawal syndrome.

Summary and future directions

It is crucial that patients with alcohol withdrawal syndrome receive appropriate and sufficient treatment in a timely manner. Alcohol withdrawal syndrome is a potentially life-threatening condition, and if it is left untreated, mild to moderate forms can progress to more severe conditions. For example, delirium tremens is almost always the result of no treatment or not enough treatment.[2] Even in less severe forms, alcohol withdrawal syndrome is a major source of distress and makes it difficult for people who experience withdrawal symptoms to stop drinking.

Moreover, several studies have shown that alcohol withdrawal syndrome negatively affects the human brain structure and function. Repeated episodes of alcohol withdrawal syndrome can damage the neurons and has negative impacts on a patient's autonomic, cognitive, and emotional function.[46,47]

Although benzodiazepines are the cornerstone of drug treatment for alcohol withdrawal syndrome, their use usually causes unwanted side effects, and it is essential to study other potential options with a better safety profile. Treatment with benzodiazepine drugs, especially in people who drink alcohol, may cause too much sedation, slow breathing, retard psychomotor movement, and impair cognitive processes. Benzodiazepines are typically metabolized through the liver and have drug-drug interactions with many other drugs.

Therefore, patients with liver disease and those who take other medications are at increased risk for developing serious side effects. Benzodiazepines' addictive properties[48] are another limiting factor in their use in people who already have a substance use disorder.

While more research is needed, the studies summarized in this chapter suggest that baclofen can be considered a promising medication for the treatment of alcohol withdrawal syndrome. Treatment with baclofen reduced the severity of uncomplicated withdrawal symptoms in both animal and human studies. Compared with benzodiazepines, baclofen has few side effects and no reported addictive properties, making it a more favorable drug in clinical practice. Baclofen is an easily manageable drug; has a wide safety margin; and can be prescribed in outpatient settings, which significantly decreases the cost of care in contrast to hospitalization. No pleasant effects or cravings for the drug have been reported in baclofen-treated patients; therefore, people are not vulnerable to abuse the drug or become dependent after baclofen use. Previous studies have found no drug interactions between alcohol and baclofen. The fact that baclofen is not metabolized through the liver is another advantage given the high probability of liver disease in many patients with alcohol use disorder.

In addition to relieving withdrawal symptoms, baclofen helps people stay sober because it significantly reduces alcohol craving and drinking, according to various studies (see Chapter 3). This is particularly important because using a single medication such as baclofen, which targets different aspects of alcohol dependence (including craving, drinking, and withdrawal) would not only be helpful in the short term but could also help patients successfully complete a long-term treatment program.

In some patients, withdrawal symptoms persist for months after detoxification (that is, "protracted alcohol withdrawal syndrome"),[2] highlighting an important role for baclofen's anti-anxiety effects[33,49] and preventive capacity[39] in preventing relapse in the long term. Therefore, compared with benzodiazepines, which are usually used for short-term symptomatic therapy, baclofen could be considered an option for long-term maintenance treatment.

However, in spite of the advantages mentioned previously and the fact that baclofen seems to be safe and effective in reducing withdrawal symptoms, it is important to remember that benzodiazepines remain the gold standard of treatment for alcohol withdrawal syndrome. Benzodiazepines have been studied in many well-designed studies and are the only class of medications with proven effectiveness in reducing the risk of alcohol withdrawal syndrome complications (seizures and delirium tremens).

Baclofen has been tested as a treatment for alcohol withdrawal in just a few studies with a small number of subjects, and no data exist regarding its effectiveness in complicated forms. The current evidence is promising, but it is not enough[50] and, until further studies are done, benzodiazepines should not be replaced by baclofen for treating alcohol withdrawal syndrome. However, baclofen's ability to reduce the need for benzodiazepines seems important, and if confirmed in future studies, add-on therapy with baclofen may become a promising and complementary approach for the management of alcohol withdrawal syndrome.

More studies are needed to draw conclusions about the possible role of baclofen in relation to alcohol withdrawal syndrome. The controversial effects of baclofen on seizures (whether it promotes or prevents convulsions),[30,32,51] the cost-effectiveness of baclofen treatment compared with that of benzodiazepines,[52] and finding the appropriate dosage and route of administration (for example, by mouth or shot) are just a few examples of questions that need to be addressed in this regard.

In conclusion, baclofen seems to be a promising drug for the treatment of alcohol withdrawal syndrome. However, more well-designed, randomized, controlled trials are needed to further investigate its safety and effectiveness.

Acknowledgments

The authors would like to thank Karen Smith (National Institutes of Health Library) for proofreading and bibliographic support, and Andrew S. Aston (Section on Clinical Psychoneuroendocrinology and Neuropsychopharmacology, National Institute on Alcohol Abuse and Alcoholism and National Institute on Drug Abuse, National Institutes of Health) for technical assistance. This work was supported by the National Institutes of Health intramural funding (Grant #ZIA-AA000218, Section on Clinical Psychoneuroendocrinology and Neuropsychopharmacology; principal investigator: Lorenzo Leggio), jointly supported by the National Institute on Alcohol Abuse and Alcoholism Division of Intramural Clinical and Biological Research and the National Institute on Drug Abuse Intramural Research Program.

References

1. Hall W, Zador D. The alcohol withdrawal syndrome. *Lancet.* 1997;349(9069):1897-900.
2. McKeon A, Frye MA, Delanty N. The alcohol withdrawal syndrome. *J Neurol Neurosurg Psychiatry.* 2008;79(8):854-62.
3. Mirijello A, D'Angelo C, Ferrulli A, et al. Identification and management of alcohol withdrawal syndrome. *Drugs.* 2015;75(4):353-65.
4. Bard MR, Goettler CE, Toschlog EA, et al. Alcohol withdrawal syndrome: Turning minor injuries into a major problem. *J Trauma.* 2006;61(6):1441-5; discussion 5-6.
5. Dissanaike S, Halldorsson A, Frezza EE, Griswold J. An ethanol protocol to prevent alcohol withdrawal syndrome. *J Am Coll Surg.* 2006;203(2):186-91.
6. Schuckit MA. Recognition and management of withdrawal delirium (delirium tremens). *N Engl J Med.* 2014;371(22):2109-13.
7. Erwin WE, Williams DB, Speir WA. Delirium tremens. *SMJ.* 1998;91(5):425-32.
8. Lerner WD, Fallon HJ. The alcohol withdrawal syndrome. *N Engl J Med.* 1985;313(15):951-2.
9. Pieninkeroinen IP, Telakivi TM, Hillbom ME. Outcome in subjects with alcohol-provoked seizures. *Alcohol Clin Exp Res.* 1992;16(5):955-9.
10. Diagnostic and Statistical Manual of Mental Disorders (DSM-5®). American Psychiatric Association Publishing; 2013.
11. Petroff OA. GABA and glutamate in the human brain. *Neuroscientist.* 2002;8(6):562-73.
12. Davis KM, Wu JY. Role of glutamatergic and GABAergic systems in alcoholism. *J Biomed Sci.* 2001;8(1):7-19.
13. Chastain G. Alcohol, neurotransmitter systems, and behavior. *J Gen Psychol.* 2006;133(4):329-35.
14. Littleton J. Neurochemical mechanisms underlying alcohol withdrawal. *Alcohol Health Res World.* 1998;22(1):13-24.
15. O'Connor PG, Schottenfeld RS. Patients with alcohol problems. *N Engl J Med.* 1998;338(9):592-602.
16. Saitz R. Clinical practice. Unhealthy alcohol use. *N Engl J Med.* 2005;352(6):596-607.
17. Naranjo CA, Sellers EM, Chater K, Iversen P, Roach C, Sykora K. Nonpharmacologic intervention in acute alcohol withdrawal. *Clin Pharmacol Ther.* 1983;34(2):214-9.
18. Mayo-Smith MF. Pharmacological management of alcohol withdrawal. A meta-analysis and evidence-based practice guideline. American Society of Addiction Medicine Working Group on Pharmacological Management of Alcohol Withdrawal. *JAMA.* 1997;278(2):144-51.
19. Amato L, Minozzi S, Vecchi S, Davoli M. Benzodiazepines for alcohol withdrawal. *Cochrane Database Syst Rev.* 2010(3):CD005063.
20. Kosten TR, O'Connor PG. Management of drug and alcohol withdrawal. *N Engl J Med.* 2003;348(18):1786-95.
21. Ross HE. Benzodiazepine use and anxiolytic abuse and dependence in treated alcoholics. *Addiction.* 1993;88(2):209-18.

22. Sachdeva A, Choudhary M, Chandra M. Alcohol withdrawal syndrome: benzo-diazepines and beyond. *J Clin Diagn Res*. 2015;9(9):VE01-VE7.
23. Leggio L, Kenna GA, Swift RM. New developments for the pharmacological treatment of alcohol withdrawal syndrome. A focus on non-benzodiazepine GABAergic medications. *Prog Neuropsychopharmacol Biol Psychiatry*. 2008;32(5):1106-17.
24. Johnson BA, Swift RM, Addolorato G, Ciraulo DA, Myrick H. Safety and efficacy of GABAergic medications for treating alcoholism. *Alcohol Clin Exp Res*. 2005;29(2):248-54.
25. Hudgson P, Weightman D. Baclofen in the treatment of spasticity. *Br Med J*. 1971;4(5778):15-7.
26. Colombo G, Agabio R, Carai MA, et al. Ability of baclofen in reducing alcohol intake and withdrawal severity: I—Preclinical evidence. *Alcohol Clin Exp Res*. 2000;24(1):58-66.
27. Tarika JS, Winger G. The effects of ethanol, phenobarbital, and baclofen on ethanol withdrawal in the rhesus monkey. *Psychopharmacology* (Berl). 1980;70(2):201-8.
28. File SE, Zharkovsky A, Gulati K. Effects of baclofen and nitrendipine on ethanol withdrawal responses in the rat. *Neuropharmacology*. 1991;30(2):183-90.
29. File SE, Zharkovsky A, Hitchcott PK. Effects of nitrendipine, chlordiazepoxide, flumazenil, and baclofen on the increased anxiety resulting from alcohol withdrawal. *Prog Neuropsychopharmacol Biol Psychiatry*. 1992;16(1):87-93.
30. Humeniuk RE, White JM, Ong J. The effects of GABAB ligands on alcohol withdrawal in mice. *Pharmacol Biochem Behav*. 1994;49(3):561-6.
31. Lal H, Harris CM, Benjamin D, Springfield AC, Bhadra S, Emmett-Oglesby MW. Characterization of a pentylenetetrazol-like interoceptive stimulus produced by ethanol withdrawal. *J Pharmacol Exp Ther*. 1988;247(2):508-18.
32. Frye GD, McCown TJ, Breese GR, Peterson SL. GABAergic modulation of inferior colliculus excitability: role in the ethanol withdrawal audiogenic seizures. *J Pharmacol Exp Ther*. 1986;237(2):478-85.
33. Knapp DJ, Overstreet DH, Breese GR. Baclofen blocks expression and sensitization of anxiety-like behavior in an animal model of repeated stress and ethanol withdrawal. *Alcohol Clin Exp Res*. 2007;31(4):582-95.
34. Becker HC. Kindling in alcohol withdrawal. *Alcohol Health Res World*. 1998;22(1):25-33.
35. De Witte P, Pinto E, Ansseau M, Verbanck P. Alcohol and withdrawal: from animal research to clinical issues. *Neurosci Biobehav Rev*. 2003;27(3):189-97.
36. Sullivan JT, Sykora K, Schneiderman J, Naranjo CA, Sellers EM. Assessment of alcohol withdrawal: the revised clinical institute withdrawal assessment for alcohol scale (CIWA-Ar). *Br J Addict*. 1989;84(11):1353-7.
37. Addolorato G, Caputo F, Capristo E, et al. Rapid suppression of alcohol withdrawal syndrome by baclofen. *Am J Med*. 2002;112(3):226-9.
38. Addolorato G, Leggio L, Abenavoli L, DeLorenzi G, Parente A, Caputo F, et al. Suppression of alcohol delirium tremens by baclofen administration: a case report. *Clin Neuropharmacol*. 2003;26(5):258-62.
39. Stallings W, Schrader S. Baclofen as prophylaxis and treatment for alcohol withdrawal: a retrospective chart review. *J Okla State Med Assoc*. 2007;100(9):354-60.

40. Bostwick JM, Seaman JS. Hospitalized patients and alcohol: who is being missed? *Gen Hosp Psychiatry*. 2004;26(1):59-62.
41. Sullivan JT, Sykora K, Schneiderman J, Naranjo CA, Sellers EM. Assessment of alcohol withdrawal: the revised clinical institute withdrawal assessment for alcohol scale (CIWA-Ar). *Br J Addict*. 1989;84(11):1353-7.
42. Mirijello A, D'Angelo C, Ferrulli A, Vassallo G, Antonelli M, Caputo F, et al. Identification and management of alcohol withdrawal syndrome. *Drugs*. 2015;75(4):353-65.
43. Addolorato G, Leggio L, Abenavoli L, Agabio R, Caputo F, Capristo E, et al. Baclofen in the treatment of alcohol withdrawal syndrome: a comparative study vs diazepam. *Am J Med*. 2006;119(3):276 e13-8.
44. Lyon JE, Khan RA, Gessert CE, Larson PM, Renier CM. Treating alcohol withdrawal with oral baclofen: a randomized, double-blind, placebo-controlled trial. *J Hosp Med*. 2011;6(8):469-74.
45. Daeppen JB, Gache P, Landry U, Sekera E, Schweizer V, Gloor S, et al. Symptom-triggered vs fixed-schedule doses of benzodiazepine for alcohol withdrawal: a randomized treatment trial. *Arch Intern Med*. 2002;162(10):1117-21.
46. Kalant H. Alcohol withdrawal syndromes in the human: comparison with animal models. *Adv Exp Med Biol*. 1977;85B:57-64.
47. Duka T, Gentry J, Malcolm R, Ripley TL, Borlikova G, Stephens DN, et al. Consequences of multiple withdrawals from alcohol. *Alcohol Clin Exp Res*. 2004;28(2):233-46.
48. Licata SC, Rowlett JK. Abuse and dependence liability of benzodiazepine-type drugs: GABA(A) receptor modulation and beyond. *Pharmacol Biochem Behav*. 2008;90(1):74-89.
49. Flannery BA, Garbutt JC, Cody MW, et al. Baclofen for alcohol dependence: a preliminary open-label study. *Alcohol Clin Exp Res*. 2004;28(10):1517-23.
50. Liu J, Wang LN. Baclofen for alcohol withdrawal. *Cochrane Database Syst Rev*. 2015;4:CD008502.
51. Terrence CF, Fromm GH, Roussan MS. Baclofen. Its effect on seizure frequency. *Arch Neurol*. 1983;40(1):28-9.
52. Reddy VK, Girish K, Lakshmi P, Vijendra R, Kumar A, Harsha R. Cost-effectiveness analysis of baclofen and chlordiazepoxide in uncomplicated alcohol-withdrawal syndrome. *Indian J Pharmacol*. 2014;46(4):372-7.

Chapter Five

Baclofen Side Effects and How to Manage Them

Philippe Jaury, MD, Department of General Practice, Paris Descartes University, Sorbonne Paris Cité, Paris, France

Like all drugs that affect the mind, emotions, or behavior, baclofen has side effects. Most side effects are benign and well tolerated. However, some can be troublesome, and several can be severe. They are also unpredictable. As a general rule, they tend to become less intense and even disappear over time.

Fortunately, these side effects, which have been well known for a long time,[1] can be treated, and experienced doctors and their patients (on some very active Internet forums all over the world[2,3]) have developed ways to reduce or even eliminate most of them.

Ways to reduce baclofen side effects

Baclofen is always started with very low doses, which are increased until the effective dose is reached. This slow progression is necessary for two reasons. First, the effective dose differs from one patient to the next, and there is no way to predict the response. Second, gradually increasing the dose lessens side effects.

If a side effect does occur, there are many ways to manage it. Patients and their doctors should discuss these options to find the best one for them:

- Continue the treatment while increasing the dose. This is a good option for very motivated patients who can tolerate the side effects, at least temporarily.
- Remain at the same dose longer before increasing it again. The usual dose-adjustment step lasts 3 days, but it can be prolonged without a problem.
- Reduce the dose.
- Take the total daily dose differently over the day, and adjust the dose time schedule as recommended by the doctor.
- Take an additional medication that can help reduce the symptoms.

- The patient may want to consider taking disability leave from work to have time to deal with the symptoms.
- If a side effect is serious or intolerable, stop the baclofen treatment.

Common side effects

Common side effects have an occurrence of more than 10%.[4-6] And when they do occur, they sometimes can be severe to the point of being disabling. Patients should be sure to tell their doctor if they are troubled with any of these side effects.

Sleepiness

Sleepiness, which tends to diminish over time, is the most common side effect. Most patients can tolerate this side effect when at home but may find it difficult to manage it at work. Patients who are experiencing sleepiness should not operate motor vehicles. Patients who remain active throughout the day tend to feel less sleepy than those who do not; however, the sleepiness tends to return at rest.

Some patients also sleep badly at night; in this case, a doctor may decide to prescribe a sleep aid. If a patient drinks only after 6 p.m. or after work, he or she should take the baclofen before then (at 3 p.m. and 5 p.m.) and not take any in the morning or at lunch; doing this can help avoid sleepiness while at work. However, if patients tend to think about alcohol in the morning, they should take the baclofen in the morning, but at a lower dose. Doctors can advise their patients on what practice might be best for them.

Because people with alcoholism often lack certain vitamins, a doctor may suggest taking vitamins, amino acids, and micronutrients to increase alertness. He or she may also recommend drinking coffee or other caffeinated drinks to stay alert at work.

Weakness and lack of energy

Weakness and lack of energy are often linked to sleepiness and sleep disorders; they also can be a symptom of depression. They occur most often when patients drink alcohol while taking baclofen. That is, it is possible to continue to occasionally drink alcohol with baclofen; women can have up to 0.7 ounces, and men can have 1.4 ounces. Weakness and lack of energy often improve over time on their own.

Insomnia and sleep disturbances

Some patients complain of problems with falling asleep during the day; in this case, a doctor may recommend or prescribe a sleep aid to take before bed. If the patient awakes repeatedly during the night and is tired in the morning, longer-acting sleep aids may be needed.

Note that, like marijuana, alcohol is sometimes used as a sleep aid; however, alcohol only interferes with sleep. Stopping alcohol use can therefore cause sleep disorders that are not necessarily linked to baclofen. In fact, many patients sleep much better with baclofen because their muscles are much more relaxed and they are much less anxious.

Sleep apnea, a condition in which people stop breathing many times during sleep, causing them to wake up, also disturbs sleep. Baclofen is not linked with sleep apnea. Patients should not hesitate to ask their doctor for a sleep study to check for sleep apnea if they are overweight, have high blood pressure, or their sleep partner reports that they snore or otherwise have altered breathing patterns during sleep.

Pain or numbness in the arms or legs

Some patients have pain with numbness or sensations such as "pins and needles" in the arms or legs. These side effects occur most often at night and can be disabling. These sensations tend to affect the arms most often. Some patients may require high doses of vitamin B to improve; if that fails, the dose of baclofen may need to be reduced or stopped. Stopping baclofen results in swift resolution of these side effects.

Tinnitus

Tinnitus, or permanent ringing or whistling in the ears, can occur in one or both ears. If a patient had tinnitus before starting baclofen, the drug may worsen it. Doctors should rule out vascular problems and high blood pressure. Nondrug treatments may help should the tinnitus become disabling.

Headache

Headaches can occur with baclofen use, usually in the morning. They tend to affect the whole head, sometimes with throbbing pain. However, they generally disappear during the day, and an over-the-counter painkiller is usually the only treatment that is needed.

Depressed mood

Depressed patients sometimes use alcohol as an anesthetic to avoid facing a difficult reality. Moreover, alcohol use can cause or worsen depression. Likewise, quitting drinking can lead to depression in patients who become aware of their failures and mistakes and of how they have hurt those around them with their behaviors.

Baclofen has not been shown to cause depression. However, if a patient is or becomes depressed, he or she should see a doctor right away; the doctor may decide to prescribe an antidepressant medication to help reduce those symptoms. Also, some patients report that the combination of baclofen and stopping alcohol enables them to be less sensitive and reactive to other people's actions and turns of events, which helps them lift their mood.

Nausea

Some patients report nausea when starting baclofen; however, the nausea usually disappears when the baclofen dose is increased. Until then, a doctor can give the patient a prescription for a medication to help relieve the nausea.

Vertigo and dizziness

Patients taking baclofen sometimes feel as if they are about to fall, which they compare to the feeling of instability they had when they drank too much. This side effect can be uncomfortable. In this case, a doctor may choose to either keep the patient on the same baclofen dose until the feelings of instability pass or reduce the dose.

Concentration problems

Problems with concentration are almost always linked to sleepiness and fatigue. Time usually reduces these side effects, and they rarely cause patients to stop treatment. Problems with memory are more strongly linked to alcohol-associated brain damage than to baclofen.

Sweating

This side effect, which is typically worse at night, can be very bothersome. Some experts think it is linked to withdrawal from alcohol and baclofen and recommend 20 mg of baclofen at bedtime. If this does not work, a doctor may prescribe a drug that can reduce the sweating.

Muscle weakness

Muscle weakness is often related to fatigue, and it can be disabling in people whose job requires them to perform manual labor. In this case, it may be necessary to increase the dosage of baclofen more slowly, which usually helps resolve this side effect.

Less common side effects

While these side effects are less common, they can be just as serious and disabling and can require a doctor's care.

Baclofen withdrawal syndrome with a confused state

Baclofen must never be stopped abruptly. As with abrupt withdrawal from alcohol in alcohol-dependent patients, the sudden withdrawal of baclofen (at doses higher than 120 mg) can cause a syndrome with a confused state or even delirium tremens. For this reason, some alcohol specialists[6] say that baclofen may be a substitution product, much as the drug methadone is for heroin. Hospitalization is necessary in these cases.

On occasion, confused states occur with baclofen alone or in combination with other medications such as anti-anxiety drugs or even with alcohol. A reduced dose of baclofen and stopping of other drugs that affect the mind, emotions, or behavior usually resolves this side effect.

Hallucinations

Hallucinations (seeing or hearing things that are not there) are anxiety inducing and justify a reduction in the baclofen dose. In psychotic patients, an increase of the dose of anti-psychotic medication may be needed as well.

Swelling of the legs and hands

In rare cases, the muscle relaxant effect of baclofen can produce swollen legs and even hands, especially in women. Wearing support stockings is generally all that is needed to resolve the problem in the legs.

Hypomania and excitation

Although rare, hypomania (over-excitation) can occur with the use of baclofen. If a patient is in an unusually good mood and does not need sleep, is agitated, uninhibited, and extremely talkative, he or she may be in a hypo-manic state. Hypomania can occur in patients who have never experienced it before. In most patients, hypomania is not harmful and disappears in time.

However, for this reason, people who have bipolar disorder (also known as manic depression) should not take baclofen unless their doctor recom-mends it. If a patient experiences these symptoms, he or she should see a doc-tor right away. He or she may either reduce the dose of baclofen or stop the treatment altogether. The patient may also be referred to a psychiatrist, who may prescribe a mood-regulating medication.

Conclusions and future directions

Although the great majority of side effects are known and can be managed with or without medication, the results of double-blinded, placebo-controlled clinical studies (neither the patient nor the doctor knows whether the patient is receiving the active drug or the placebo) help us better understand which side effects are due to baclofen and which are due to other factors.

No significant link has been found between patient characteristics and the onset of side effects. However, current genetic baclofen studies may help identify what kind of people benefit most from baclofen with the fewest side effects. This information could help doctors better tailor the dose and dose time schedule for each patient as well as better predict which side effects are most likely to occur. The availability of new formulations for doctors with new doses will help them prescribe effective dosages of baclofen that can help reduce or eliminate some side effects.

References
1.   Smith CR, LaRocca NG, Giesser BS, et al. High-dose oral baclofen: experience in patients with multiple sclerosis. *Neurology*. 1991 Nov;41(11):1829-31.
2.   Forum alcool, alcoolisme et autres addictions: Alcoolisme et baclofène (in French). Available at: www.baclofene.com. Accessed January 13, 2016.
3.   Baclofene: Forum baclofène du réseau AUBES (in French). Available at: www.baclofene.fr. Accessed January 13, 2016.
4.   Gache P, de Beaurepaire R, Jaury P, Jousseaume B, Rapp A, de la Selle P. Pre-scribing guide for baclofen in the treatment of alcoholism for use by physicians. *Br J Med Medical Res*. 2013;4(5):1164-74.
5.   Rigal L, Legay Huang L, et al. Tolerability of high-dose baclofen in the treat-ment of patients with alcohol disorders: a retrospective study. *Alcohol*.

2015;50(5):551-7.

6. Müller CA, Geisel O, Pelz P, Higl V,Krüger J, Stickel A, Beck A, Wernecke KD,
    Hellweg R, Heinz A. High-dose baclofen for the treatment of alcohol depen-
    dence (BACLAD study): A randomized, placebo-controlled trial. *Eur Neuropsy-
    chopharmacol.* 2015;25(8):1167-77.

Glossary

Absence seizures: A seizure consisting of a "staring out into space" in which the affected person is not responsive or aware of his or her surroundings.

Acamprosate: A medication used in the treatment of alcohol dependence. It is believed to stabilize the balance of neurotransmitters in the brain that would otherwise be upset by withdrawal from alcohol.

Aerophagia: Excessive, usually unconscious, swallowing of air caused by anxiety.

Agitation: Racing of thoughts and purposeless restlessness caused by anxiety.

Alcohol abstinence: Refraining from the use of alcohol.

Alcohol abuse: Misuse or excessive intake of alcohol.

Alcoholics Anonymous: An international group of recovering alcoholics who work to become and stay sober through abstinence, meetings, and a 12-step program.

Alcoholism: A pattern of alcohol abuse that negatively affects a person's social, cognitive, and occupational functioning. Also called alcohol use disorder.

Aldosterone: A hormone secreted by the adrenal cortex that promotes the retention of sodium, bicarbonate, and water and the excretion of hydrogen ions and potassium.

Alcohol use disorder: See *alcoholism*.

Alcohol withdrawal syndrome: A potentially life-threatening series of signs and symptoms that occurs after the cessation of alcohol used to the point of intoxication. Symptoms may range from heavy sweating, agitation, and an inability to sleep to hallucinations and seizures.

Amino acids: The building blocks of protein that also have a role in metabolism.

Ataxia: A lack of control over the muscles during voluntary movements such as walking.

Antidepressants: Drugs designed to relieve depression.

Anxiety: An unpleasant feeling that bad things are about to happen. Symptoms can include sweating, tremors, increased heart rate, weakness, and fatigue.

Baclofen: A drug given orally for the treatment of spasticity in cases of multiple sclerosis, spinal cord diseases, and spinal cord injury. It is also sometimes prescribed off-label for the treatment of alcoholism.

Baseline: A set of observations or data that are used as a comparison or control.

Benign: Not harmful.

Benzodiazepines: A class of drugs that works on the central nervous system, specifically on GABA-A receptors in the brain. Also known as tranquilizers.

Bias: A systematic error in study design that skews study results.

Binge-eating disorder: See *bulimia nervosa*.

Bipolar disorder: A mood disorder in which episodes of depression alternate with episodes of mania or hypomania. Also called manic depression.

Borderline personality disorder: A disorder marked by unstable mood, self-image, and relationships. Symptoms also include self-harming behaviors, uncontrolled outbursts of anger, paranoia, threats of suicide, and dissociation.

Bulimia nervosa: A pattern of binging on food and then vomiting meant to promote weight loss or prevent weight gain.

Cannabinoids: Marijuana-derived medications.

Case report: A detailed report on an individual patient, including signs and symptoms, diagnosis, treatment, and follow up.

Cirrhosis: Scarring of the liver due to diseases or conditions such as alcohol use disorder.

Compassionate use: Prescribing a drug unapproved for a particular condition for seriously ill patients who have no other effective treatment options.

Complications: Another health condition that aggravates the already existing one.

Compulsive: Resulting from an irresistible urge.

Concurrent: Occurring at the same time.

Control group: A group that is not a part of the experiment in which an independent variable is being tested. It is used for purposes of comparison.

Convulsions: Sudden involuntary movements of a limb or other part of the body.

Cortisol: A steroid hormone produced in response to stress. It is also used as a medication known as hydrocortisone.

Creatinine: A waste product produced by the muscle and by meat in the diet. The rate at which creatinine clears the body in the urine is a marker of kidney health because kidneys filter creatinine from the blood. Therefore, a creatinine clearance test can show how well the kidneys are working.

Data set: A group of data that can be manipulated by a computer.

Delirium tremens: A set of severe signs and symptoms that can occur after alcohol withdrawal, usually within 48 to 96 hours after the last drink; however, symptoms can emerge up to 10 days afterward. Signs and symptoms can include seizures, trembling, changes in the ability to think, agitation, irritability, confusion, delirium, fear, hallucinations, restlessness, fatigue, depression, loss of appetite, nausea, heart palpitations, sweating, chest pain, fever, and stomach pain.

Delusions: Belief in something that is not based in reality.

Dependence: A physical reliance on alcohol, drugs, or other substances to achieve a feeling of well-being, alertness, or relaxation.

Depression: A common, serious mood disorder consisting of persistent feelings of sadness, worthlessness, thoughts of self-harm, guilt, shame, hopelessness, and disinterest in normally pleasurable activities. There are many kinds of depression, some of which include psychosis, or a break from reality consisting of delusions or hallucinations.

Detoxification: Excretion or removal of alcohol or other harmful substances from the body.

Diabetes: An umbrella term for several diseases that affect how the body uses blood glucose (sugar). In type 1 diabetes, or childhood diabetes, the pancreas stops making insulin, and as a result, glucose can build up to dangerous levels in the blood. In type 2 diabetes, either the pancreas makes too little insulin, or the body cannot use the insulin effectively.

Disinhibition: An absence of restraint that shows itself as a disregard for normally accepted behavior, impulsivity, and impaired evaluation of risk.

Disulfiram: A drug given to people with alcoholism, disulfiram causes unpleasant effects not unlike that of a hangover when the person drinks any amount of alcohol. The effects include anxiety, confusion, flushing of the face, headache, nausea, chest pain, sweating, and breathing problems. The drug is meant to deter the person from drinking alcohol.

Dopamine: A neurotransmitter produced by the brain that affects the brain's reward and well-being centers.

Dosage: The amount and timing of a drug to be taken regularly over a period of time.

Dose: The amount of a drug to be taken at one time.

Double-blind: A study in which neither the researchers nor the participants know who is receiving the study drug.

Encephalopathy: Brain disease, damage, or dysfunction leading to an altered mental state.

End point: The outcomes that the researchers set out to measure, compare, and report.

Epilepsy: A neurological disorder characterized by seizures and other health problems.

Ethyl alcohol: Ethanol, or a primary alcohol that is clear, colorless, and flammable that can result in acute intoxication. It is the primary type of alcohol in alcoholic beverages.

Euphoria: Intense feelings of well-being, delight, and excitement.

GABA: A transmitter responsible for inhibition in the central nervous system.

GABA-B receptors: The targets of drugs that result in muscle relaxation or work to fight addiction.

Gastro-esophageal reflux disease (GERD): A chronic digestive disease characterized by the washing back of stomach acid into the esophagus. Also called heartburn.

Genetic: Hereditary, or capable of being passed on from generation to generation.

Genotype: A person's genetic makeup, which determines things such as appearance.

GHB: A neurotransmitter and an anesthetic drug known as the "date rape drug." GHB, or gamma-hydroxybutyric acid, has been used as a treatment for alcoholism and other disorders.

Gluten: The proteins found in grains such as wheat, rye, oats, and barley. People with celiac disease have an abnormal immune response to gluten.

Half-life: The time that elapses between when a drug is taken and when it is present in the body in only half of its initial amount.

Hallucination: The perception that something is real when it is, in fact, not present.

Harm reduction: The practice of drinking less alcohol to produce less harm to the person's health and environment.

Hemiplegia: Paralysis that occurs on only one side of the body.

Hepatitis C: A liver disease caused by the hepatitis C virus. It spreads through contact with infected blood, sharing hypodermic needles, or being accidentally stuck by an infected needle. Symptoms can range from none to fever, nausea, dark-colored urine, joint pain, jaundice, fatigue, and lack of appetite.

Hormones: A group of chemical messengers excreted by the endocrine system that control most major functions of the body.

Hyperammonemia: A condition characterized by too much ammonia in the blood.

Hypomania: Low-level mania, or euphoria. Hypomania is typically benign.

Huffing: Sniffing household products such as glue, aerosol sprays, paint, and lighter fuel to "get high," or feel euphoric.

Incontinence: Accidental leakage of the bladder or bowels.

Indifference: Unconcern, apathy, or a lack of interest in a situation that would otherwise spark interest or cause worry or apprehension.

Insomnia: A common sleep disorder in which it is difficult to fall asleep and stay asleep. It can also involve early-morning awakening with an inability to get back to sleep.

Kindling: The worsening of alcohol withdrawal symptoms over repeated withdrawals from alcohol.

Lapse: A lapse represents any episode of alcohol consumption not classified as relapse.

Levodopa: The gold-standard drug for the treatment of Parkinson's disease, it is converted to the neurotransmitter dopamine in the brain.

Mania: A state of overexcitability, euphoria, grandiosity, irritability, a decreased need for sleep, racing thoughts, and elevated energy.

Medical indemnity insurance: A type of insurance plan that reimburses the policy holder or healthcare provider a predetermined amount of money, regardless of the actual costs, for certain procedures.

Mesolimbic dopamine neurons: Nerve cells involved in the mediation of alcohol intake and reinforcement.

Meta-analysis: The combination of data from multiple studies using statistical procedures.

Microdialysis: A minimally invasive sampling technique.

Micronutrient: A nutrient required in only trace amounts for good health, well-being, and normal development.

Model: An example to copy or use for comparison.

Monosodium glutamate: Also known as MSG, it is a food preservative and flavoring consisting of a sodium salt of glutamate, a nonessential amino acid.

Mood stabilizers: Antidepressant or anti-psychotic drugs used to treat and prevent mania or depression.

Nalmefene: A drug to help people with alcoholism reduce the amount of alcohol they drink by reducing the desire to drink. It is also used to reverse the effects of narcotic drugs or overdose.

Naltrexone: A drug used to prevent people with alcoholism or who abuse opiate drugs from drinking or taking the drugs again by decreasing the desire to do so.

Nausea: A sensation of uneasiness in the stomach accompanied by an urge to vomit.

Neurologist: A doctor specializing in the treatment of diseases affecting the brain, spinal cord, and nerves.

Neuron: Nerve cell that processes and sends information through chemical and electrical signals.

Neurotransmitter: A chemical messenger that transmits messages from one neuron to another.

Norepinephrine: An organic compound that functions in the body similarly to a neurotransmitter or hormone in that it is a chemical messenger. Its primary function is to mobilize the body and brain for action.

Obsessive Compulsive Drinking Scale: A questionnaire that seeks to determine how much a person drinks and how well they are able to control their drinking.

Off-label use: Use of a drug that the authorities have not approved for the treatment of a particular condition.

Open-label: A type of clinical study in which both the researchers and the participants know what kind of medication is being given.

Opioids: Narcotic medications that produce morphine-like effects such as euphoria.

Outpatient: Care received outside of the hospital setting (for example, in a clinic).

Parkinsonism: A condition that causes the movement abnormalities seen in Parkinson's disease.

Parkinson's disease: A central nervous system disease that affects movement and may cause tremors.

Pathophysiology: Disordered physiological processes related to an injury or a disease.

Penn Alcohol Craving Scale: A questionnaire aimed at assessing a person's craving for alcohol during the previous week.

Peptic ulcer: Stomach ulcers or painful sores in the lining of the stomach or the first part of the small intestine.

Peripheral nervous system: The nervous system that does not include the brain or spinal cord.

Placebo: A pill containing no medication used in studies to compare the effects of different drugs.

Placebo effect: When a research participant believes that the placebo he or she is unknowingly taking has made him or her feel better, when it actually could have had no such effect because it contains no medication.

Plasma: The yellow-colored, liquid part of blood that holds whole blood cells in suspension.

Porphyria: A group of rare diseases in which porphyrin pigments build up in the body.

Positive airway pressure mask: The part of a machine that goes over the face to help people with disorders such as sleep apnea breathe more easily during sleep.

Prospective study: A study that follows a group of patients over time.

Psychosis: A condition in which a person's perceptions and thinking patterns are disrupted, allowing him or her to see, hear, or sense things that are not there. Also called a "break from reality."

Psychotherapy: Treatment of a mental disorder by speaking with a trained therapist, psychologist, psychiatrist, or counselor. Also called talk therapy.

Randomized, controlled trial: The gold standard of studies, a randomized, controlled trial allocates people at random to receive a clinical intervention or a placebo, standard practice, or no intervention for comparison.

Receptor: A part of a cell that can respond to an external stimulus (for example, drug, light, heat) and transmit a chemical signal to a sensory nerve.

Regimen: A prescribed course of treatment to promote health.

Reimbursement: Repayment.

Relapse: For classification purposes, relapse is defined as a daily alcohol intake of more than 4 drinks or an overall consumption of 14 drinks or more per week during at least 4 weeks.

Rumination: Regurgitation of food, or bringing food back up after swallowing it.

Schizophrenia: A serious mental illness characterized by abnormal social behavior and a break from reality (psychosis).

Sedation: A state of sleep or calm that is the result of administration of a sedative drug.

Selective serotonin reuptake inhibitors: The most commonly used antidepressant drugs, these work by increasing the availability of the neurotransmitter serotonin in the brain.

Self-mutilation: Cutting oneself to achieve psychological relief.

Serotonin: A neurotransmitter, or chemical messenger, in the brain that is believed to contribute to feelings of well-being.

Side effects: Typically unwanted and unpleasant effects of drugs that can interfere with a person's ability to tolerate the drugs or can result in illness.

Sleep apnea: A condition in which people stop breathing many times during sleep, causing them to wake up.

Spasticity: A condition in which the muscles stiffen, affecting movement or speech.

State-Trait Inventory Scale: A commonly used questionnaire used to gauge traits and anxiety in the diagnosis of anxiety.

Supragastric belching: The intentional belching of air from above the stomach related to anxiety.

Talk therapy: An ongoing conversation between a doctor and patient. There are many different kinds of talk therapy, the most common of which is cognitive behavioral therapy, in which a therapist evaluates how negative thought patterns are influencing mood and then tries to disrupt those patterns.

Tetraplegia: Partial or total paralysis of all four limbs and the torso.

Tinnitus: Permanent ringing or whistling in the ears.

Tolerance (alcohol): The increasing ability to drink larger and larger quantities of alcohol.

Tonic-clonic seizures: A convulsive seizure in which the person loses consciousness, his or her muscles stiffen, and he or she makes jerking movements.

Toxic: Poisonous, or capable of causing serious disease or death.

Tremor: Involuntary shaking, often of the hands.

Trial: Research study that evaluates the ability of new approaches to the prevention or treatment of medical disorders.

Uninhibited: Unrestrained expression of thoughts or feelings.

Urinary incontinence: The involuntary leaking of urine as a result of stress, muscle weakness, or spasms.

Vascular: Relating to blood vessels.

Vertigo: Dizziness, nausea, ringing in the ears, or a sense of spinning that is often caused by a problem with the inner ear.

Index

www.ingramcontent.com/pod-product-compliance
Lightning Source LLC
Chambersburg PA
CBHW070930270326
41927CB00011B/2795